Supporting mental wellbeing,
building emotional sustainability

I'M GETTING THERE

Overcoming emotional obstacles and
hidden patterns that can block change

Amberley Meredith M.Sc.

Registered Psychologist with over 25 years
experience in mental health

© Amberley Meredith 2025

Print copy: ISBN: 978-1-7640628-2-4
E-book: ISBN: 978-1-7640628-3-1

All rights reserved.

No part of this publication may be reproduced, stored in a retrieval system, or transmitted in any form or by any means—electronic, mechanical, photocopying, recording, or otherwise—without the prior written permission of the copyright owner, except for brief quotations used for the purposes of review, commentary, or scholarly work, with appropriate acknowledgement.

This publication is not a substitute for professional mental health advice or treatment. Readers experiencing distress are encouraged to seek support from a qualified mental health professional.

Published in Australia.

Protected under the Copyright Act 1968 (Cth) and applicable international laws.

For permissions or inquiries, visit:

www.adaptablesustainablepsychology.com

Front Cover Design: Britt Wilson

Also Available in the Adaptable Sustainable Psychology Collection:

Book 1: The Subtle Injury of Influence

*Managing experiences, people
and media that affect your mental health*

Book 2: I'm Getting There

*Overcoming emotional obstacles
and hidden patterns that can block change*

Book 3: Self-Improvement Burnout

When to start, when to stop

Book 4: Steps Towards Kindness and Accountability

The dance of healthier relationships

Dedication:

This series is dedicated to everyone who has survived: survived pain, survived trauma, survived disappointment.

Your stories are the true history of human culture, and an integral part of our evolution.

About the Author:

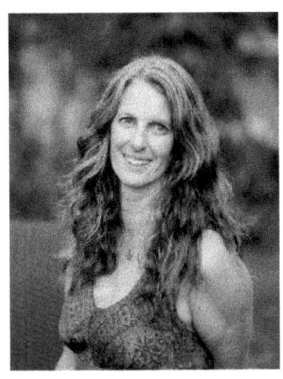
Amberley Meredith has worked in the field of mental health and wellbeing for over 25 years. Her professional journey began in 1995 as a volunteer in a UK-based drug and alcohol drop-in centre. She went on to complete a Bachelor of Science in Psychology and a Master of Science in Health Psychology in the United Kingdom.

Amberley has been registered as a psychologist in both Australia and New Zealand for over 20 years. Across her career, she has worked in diverse settings including acute mental health care and working as an authorised officer, held roles in community mental health services and on a children's acquired brain injury team, run a regional eating disorder liaison service, and worked with numerous multidisciplinary teams. She has continued to operate her own clinic in private practice across most of her career, specialising more in trauma and disability for the past decade. She has designed and facilitated trauma-informed retreats and created psycho-educational programs for community and corporate environments.

Drawing on over 60,000 hours of professional practice with individuals, couples, and groups, Amberley created this self-development series to share practical strategies derived from evidence-based psychological approaches. Her work integrates knowledge from a range of therapeutic frameworks and psychology principles.

Amberley is committed to making psychological knowledge accessible and meaningful. Her educational resources are designed to support reflection, insight, and the development of emotional wellbeing in an inclusive, relatable way. Amberley is continually inspired by what people can achieve when vulnerability is met with self-belief.

Adaptable Sustainable Psychology Disclaimer:

This content is intended for general educational and informational purposes only. It is not a substitute for professional psychological advice, diagnosis, or treatment. If you are experiencing distress or mental health concerns, please consult a registered psychologist or qualified healthcare provider.

The concepts and tools described in this series are based on psychological theory and practice but are not intended to represent or replace personalised therapeutic support. Outcomes may vary based on individual circumstances.

The exercises and questions provided are for educational and self-reflective purposes only. If at any point you feel distressed, overwhelmed, or emotionally unsettled while completing these exercises or responding to the questions, please seek support from a qualified mental health professional. This material is not a substitute for therapy or clinical intervention.

Amberley Meredith is a registered psychologist with the Australian Health Practitioner Regulation Agency (AHPRA). Her registration prohibits offering testimonials or making claims of guaranteed outcomes.

Contents

Welcome and namaste – the divine in me honours the divine in you. 1
   Exercise: Memory Capture 14
1. Setting the Mind 16
   Exercise: Grounding-Kindness Meditation 21
   Exercise: Train Your Brain to Change 23
   Exercise: The Memory Palace 30
   Pause—Reflect—Landscape 34
2. Being Human is Not Easy 39
   Exercise: Witnessing Breathing 48
   Pause—Reflect—Landscape 50
3. Emotions as Informants 55
   Exercise: Observation and Witnessing Meditation 61
   Pause—Reflect—Landscape 64
4. Denial. It's not just a river in Africa 69
   Exercise: Your Emotional Coping Pie 78
   Pause—Reflect—Landscape 81
5. It Wasn't Me! Managing the Intrusion of Guilt and Influence of Fear 87
   Exercise: Fear and Guilt Management Protocol 99
   Pause—Reflect—Landscape 106

6. Positive Emotional Coping. 111
    Exercise: Developing Positive Emotional Management: Pause, Process, Progress. 120
    Pause—Reflect—Landscape 127

7. When Thinking Can be Bad for Your Health 133
    Exercise: Sitting with Pain Meditation 139
    Exercise: Playing with Time 142
    Pause—Reflect—Landscape 145

8. Attachment – The Sticky Tape of the Mind 151
    Exercise: Detachment of Attachment 162
    Pause—Reflect—Landscape 165

9. Review of Insights into You 168
    Exercise: Insights Gained into you 174
    Exercise: Memory Capture Revisited. 177

Next Steps 179

10. Alternative Self-Talk Tables 181

Acknowledgments - With Gratitude. 201

Welcome and namaste – the divine in me honours the divine in you.

Change can be difficult, and maintaining change over time may be even more challenging. By identifying the hidden patterns and potential obstacles that could influence our capacity to initiate and maintain change, and by considering strategies to manage these challenges, we may improve our ability to support meaningful and sustainable growth. Whether it's a fixed or set mind that's holding us back, or we're having trouble developing the kind of mindset that can overcome emotional blocks, our freedom to feel capable of change can be compromised. Some of our resistance to change may arise from the subtle influences of unconscious biases that hold us back or repeatedly land us in confirmation bias patterns, where we can conclude that no change is necessary. With fear and guilt potentially lurking in the background, our conscious efforts to grow may be unconsciously sabotaged by internal narratives that do not support us or believe in our capacity to follow through. Attaching to ideals and ideas, roles and relationships, dreams and situations can hinder and prevent us from establishing patterns of sustainable change.

With so many hidden obstacles, the relevance and importance of understanding ourselves, especially when it comes to making changes that support long-term wellbeing, becomes even more significant. While change can be initiated through insight, it is sustained through self-belief and the determination to remain kind and encouraging toward ourselves. If you haven't yet developed the ability to offer yourself compassion, worked out how to be comfortable with uncomfortable emotions or you feel emotionally compromised in being able to maintain motivation and focus, then change may feel out of reach. There are many valuable books on change, mental wellness, how to live life better, how to find love, how to keep love, increase your success and wealth. Yet many of us struggle to create changes that help to bring us those things.

With so much knowledge now available about how we work, why things hurt and what we can do to live life better, we might ask why is that? The answer is, of course, as complex as we are, it is multi-layered. Pretty much all of us have either had a personal experience of trying to change, only to be unsuccessful at implementing new habits in the long term, or we know people who have tried to change and simply returned to how they used to be. As we learnt from Book 1, change can take time and possibly a very large amount of repetition before it can become an automatic habit. Our emotional experiences, self-doubt, external distractions and even just boredom and impatience can all get in the way of creating that sustainable change. We can feel like everything around us is putting us under pressure to constantly achieve more, be more and grow more, somehow, perhaps, insinuating we are not enough without being engrossed in this seemingly endless spiral of change. The field of wellbeing often promotes ideals and ways of living that many of us aspire to. However, unless your core sense of self is already well-established, you know yourself exceptionally well, you can maintain an honest self-awareness, you've

Welcome and namaste – the divine in me honours the divine in you.

addressed most of the underlying beliefs about not being "good enough," and you're consistently managing your internal biases and the many external influences designed to sway your thoughts and behaviours, it can be challenging to achieve, let alone sustain, these aspirational ways of living.

In this era of unprecedented ease, our lives have never been so physically comfortable in many ways. But is this coinciding with declines in our general happiness? Those living in places where change unfolds more slowly can often seem much happier, perhaps smiling more easily or appearing friendlier to strangers. We're surrounded by labour-saving devices and instant-access conveniences that promise ease and speed. While these advances have created more space for us to pursue change, they can also feel never-ending, even relentlessly demanding. Have all these technological breakthroughs left us with too much time to think and feel?

It may be that, due to the way some of this technology has evolved and the easy access of commodities, we have created the very opposite of our intention, instead of using technology to grant us time and space to be free to enjoy being ourselves this has all had a narrowing effect on how we perceive things and how we think, causing us to hyperfocus on constant change and leaning into unhelpful perfectionistic attitudes that then impact how we are feeling, creating both stress and distress.

Is our ability to stop, pause, assess and critically analyse information and take in that bigger picture potentially being eroded through the fast flow of continuously changing information and the powerful prism of constant change?

How often have you had the experience of just finishing to learn how to use your new device, then another upgrade comes along. One type of food is good for you and then it's not, electric cars are going to save the planet, then we can't dispose of them once they don't work anymore. This hyper speed of change and information means that our ability to take in the bigger picture has been brought down into a small window that changes in the blink of an eye. Even one of the modern world's primary vehicles for this information, the mobile phone, may affect our visual spatial capacity and might compromise our capacity to stop and take in a wider and deeper view and look around us. Think about how often we sit on our phone and the information changes in a nano second, this small window into life that can only fit so much information on one screen. Perhaps, we have seen or been that person who walks into something because we are busy looking at our phone or tripped over our own feet whilst scrolling, not paid attention to conversations people are trying to have with us or connecting virtually more than physically, or simply been too distracted to do our chores or tasks.

The idea of labour-saving devices and the paper free world was meant to clear space for us to do other things. Yet it can feel like we spend all our time learning new things or have to get more done or have extra standards that we must comply with, where there is a space that could be occupied with just being it seems something else can always take up our focus and energy. A more meaningful way to use this time and space may be to focus on psychologically and emotionally evolving how we access, apply, and integrate change into our lives. Yet this becomes far more difficult when our cognitive and emotional capacity narrows, leaving us to address only isolated fragments of unhelpful thoughts or behaviours, or to focus on just one aspect of what we are feeling. This may be why many of the directions on how to change do not always land with us. You can use a breathing exercise to manage anxiety and have a sign on your wall that says you are enough. But if you are still using a perfectionist mindset that cares what everyone else thinks, then your improvements, whilst a great start, are not necessarily going to create the deeper change you are seeking. If you doubt your abilities, anxiety can still overwhelm you when under pressure and the breathwork is forgotten in amongst the overwhelm. You can ask someone if they feel confident and deserving. They reflect, thinking, "Yes, I feel I am worthy because I am told to believe that by the sign on my wall." But later, they start to tell you they feel lonely, even when hanging out with their friends and feel like they have nothing to offer, indicating that they clearly don't feel worthy in all aspects of their life. Somehow the work on believing you are enough has not filtered through to all domains. You could have a super fit body from going to the gym but still feel you're not as good as others and negatively compare yourself, ending up unable to be content in being you.

Having an Adaptable Sustainable Psychology (ASP) framework may help you explore how to apply broader wellbeing concepts and strategies in a way that feels relevant and achievable in your own life and helps you get into the corners not always explored.

It offers a personalised approach to support lasting change by encouraging ongoing reflection and self-awareness, and a chance to examine the multiple angles and areas that could be affecting your overall sense of wellbeing. With ASP, you're invited to explore the deeper layers of your experiences, the "why", while developing new strategies for the "how." This approach is centred on your individual needs and experiences, rather than based on someone else's outcomes, singular aspects or a list of perceived perfected ideals.

If you want to start the work of challenging what has been given to you by people, experiences, or social programming (be it the media or cultural/political system), then you might not only have to work out what would benefit from being changed, but also be prepared to go **in-depth,** be **patient** and **consistent.** These are qualities that may be hard to access sometimes in the information-rich and fast-paced world we live in. Promises of instantaneous delivery, fast food, 10 steps to riches and happiness, latest updates and more-rapid-than-ever service can all hoodwink us into being too demanding of our human brain that biologically needs time to formulate new habits and practices to make self-comfort and self-support a thing or process deep trauma or big hurts that require a lot of nurture, care and help to manage.

Have you ever had the experience of visualising a goal, desire, or future version of yourself or your life, but found it difficult to make it a reality? While our minds can imagine possibilities in an instant, aligning those visions with our emotions, behaviours, and the people around us often takes a combination of honest in-depth information on ourselves, the overcoming of emotional obstacles and the management of hidden negative thinking patterns that may require time, patience, and support. In Book 2 of the Adaptable Sustainable Psychology collection, we explore some of the common challenges that may interrupt or delay personal growth and stop you from being at peace with your progress.

This book focuses on how unseen biases and emotions can influence the change process and offers reflective practices to help you strengthen your cognitive and emotional framework from different perspectives. Through continued self-awareness and self-compassion, you may begin to cultivate a sense of being "enough" just as you are. By gently exploring your inner world, you can identify ways to support yourself in navigating life with greater alignment between your values and your actions, less shaped by external pressures and more guided by your authentic self.

I'm Getting There invites you to engage in a process of thoughtful self-reflection, gently exploring your inner world to better understand the person you are at your core, developing a positive emotional management framework for coping with those more challenging feelings and learning about any unconscious biases that may be hindering you from changing. Identifying overthinking patterns that could be derailing your best efforts, and seeing what might be holding you back from letting go of the things that could foster a sense of peace in being you and feeling more comfortable accepting new realities. The aim is to provide tools and perspectives that may support you in identifying and re-evaluating unhelpful patterns or influences that may have impacted you over time, sometimes in ways that are not immediately obvious. Rather than offering quick fixes, the Adaptable Sustainable Psychology collection encourages approaches that are designed to be emotionally sustainable, helpful in the present while also considerate of your long-term wellbeing. At its heart, this journey is about fostering a sense of contentment in being yourself, and supporting you in developing ways to respond to life that feel authentic and balanced. The foundation for this process is the development of your own Adaptable Sustainable Psychology—an approach that centres around who you are, what works for you, and how you choose to grow.

The Voyage into You – Instructions for the Journey

We provide these guidelines in each of our books to help support you and remind you of how to get the most out of the material. This work is in no way meant to replace active therapy, nor is it prescribed to fix serious psychological problems that require the support and help of a trained professional.

There are many ways that you might use this work. You may be using it on your own or as a couple. You could be a professional therapist using it with a client. You might even choose to do it with a small group of friends, or make it part of your professional organisation's wellbeing program. Whichever way you pick, take your time with it. It's designed to help you run the marathon, not win the sprint. The skills taught here take a long time to develop. By that, we do mean years. If you are seeking the quick fix then, sadly, this is not going to meet that desire. The human brain may take a very long time to integrate new ways of being into an automatic habit, it requires extensive repetition and focus, but the pay offs from staying the course could be well worth the effort. **Patience, repetition and commitment need to be your companions.**

If you're someone who has been exposed to trauma, please be gentle and patient with yourself throughout the recovery journey. You may require professional support and help from qualified therapists to fully understand all the psychological, emotional, neurological and physiological impacts of trauma. Whilst the techniques discussed throughout this collection of books have relevance to anyone who has suffered trauma, due to the potentially serious impacts on the structures of the brain, mind and body, you are advised to seek additional professional help.

Welcome and namaste – the divine in me honours the divine in you.

It is always wise to approach any therapeutic care you undertake with an attitude of being kind and gentle with yourself, knowing that extensive damage may require an extensive healing period, and just because one technique doesn't suit you, it doesn't mean there is not another pathway that might work better for you. Consider approaching your healing with a commitment to finding a way to support yourself and learning to adapt with whatever has happened, mitigating and managing the impacts, whilst finding a way to open yourself up to the joys and pleasures in life that could also be available. The powerful impact of trauma or pain may be inescapable, but the strength of your capacity to overcome it can be altered.

Take a check-in each time you pick up this book, pausing to ask yourself where your level of coping is at today. Remember, there may be areas that could be triggering and difficult. If you're feeling too busy, exhausted, or even a bit too overwhelmed, you may need to come back to it at another time. Keep doing this throughout each section, making sure you are in a receptive space to sit with what is being opened up for you. You might want to set yourself up with some quiet time. You will need pens or pencils to write with. You can write all over the book if you so wish; have fun writing in the margins! Repetition may support you in how you learn and integrate ideas and new behaviours. Reading this book once probably isn't going to lead to absorbing all the information or ideas you may find useful. Read it, reread it again, and then maybe re-read again sometime later. Keep coming back to conversations about what you have read and the insights you may experience, both in your own mind and when talking with others. This may help support and reinforce your learning.

Self-development can be an interactive and two-way

journey. Where it involves the intersections of other people's actions, thoughts, and feelings with our own. Whether they be positive or negative, and no matter where that interaction comes from, be it a person, the media, from a therapist, or even from a book, change may come from the place where we meet with someone else's ideas or views, and we consciously choose what might help us on our way to feeling better.

The exercises and questions given in these books are for educational and self-reflective purposes only. If at any point you feel distressed, overwhelmed, or emotionally unsettled while completing any of these exercises or reflecting on the questions asked, please seek support from a qualified mental health professional. This material is not a substitute for therapy or clinical intervention. The exercises are derived from a vast number of evidence-based therapies and wellbeing theories, including neuroscience, mindfulness, polyvagal theory, hope psychology, positive psychology, acceptance and commitment therapy, cognitive behavioural therapy, solution and emotion focused therapies, and psychology from a trauma-informed perspective.

The tools are likely to work differently for different kinds of people in different situations. Sometimes, a slight shift in the format works better for one person than another. There is no one kind of psychological or healing modality that fixes everything for everyone. But by working with a wide range of ideas, methods, and people, you may find the parts that resonate with you and adapt what does not. This is how you can build your psychodiversity for coping through life's challenges.

Many of the approaches discussed in this collection of books may have a more neurotypical focus but could be possibly modified to suit those coming from neurodivergent space. Remember, the information and techniques given are not about a prescription, but guidance to help you on your journey of finding what works for you and what supports you in feeling comfortable to be you. Play with the suggestions given, alter the exercises to work for you, however your brain interacts with the world, be it through a neurodivergent lens or a neurotypical one.

Alexithymia is a neuropsychological phenomenon, also known as emotional blindness, it is a personality trait that makes it difficult to experience, identify, understand, and express emotions. The term comes from Greek roots meaning "no words for emotions". Those who have alexithymia may find that they experience emotions through physical sensations, behaviours (including risk taking ones), as a somatic/bodily response (such as pain, tension, tingling) or in other unique ways, and they may find it helpful to learn to acknowledge these experiences in lieu of feeling their emotions.

If you have alexithymia, you can still work out what your signals and signs are that indicate you are having an emotional reaction or response, and you may be able to develop ways to respond to the experience. It may work for you to ameliorate emotional experiences with responses or cues such as massage, drumming, tapping, exercise, eating appropriately, or talking about the situation with a solution focused perspective. For example, if anger and hurt are expressed in risk taking behaviour such as driving too fast or wanting to hurt yourself, you could take up boxing and have a punching bag at home and when the urge to speed or hurt yourself arises divert yourself to the somewhat safer choice of using the punching bag. You could use an exercise bike to ride as fast as possible; you could run or walk as fast as possible or use a virtual reality game that requires you to fight. Anything that you feel may help you work through the emotion and safely process it.

Please also note, that as we use some guided imagery work in these books those with aphantasia, a cognitive phenomenon that describes the difficulty or inability to voluntarily create visual mental images, may need to look at pictures to help evoke the same connections or feelings.

Before you begin this journey, we invite you to please take a moment of stillness and a singular, deep breath. Bring yourself fully into this moment. Whenever you pick up this book, repeat this process so that you can check that you are ready to engage fully with what you are reading and get the most out of the material. Please remember, this book is not meant as a replacement for professional therapy. You can use it alongside a program of professional treatment or as part of your own personal growth.

1. Setting the Mind

In this section you will be learning about:

- → What is the difference between an experience and experiencing something?
- → Is yours a set mind or a mindset?
- → How the science of neuroplasticity might support the process of change.
- → Why is a flexible mind helpful for adaption?

You will need:

- ✓ If available, the work you completed on your identity and beliefs from Book 1.
- ✓ A pen and paper.
- ✓ An openness to accepting your mind might need un-setting.
- ✓ Time and space to practice a breathing exercise and complete a written exercise.
- ✓ Readiness to commit to using some of the exercises daily for at least 30 days.
- ✓ To be open to discussing your reactions, feelings, and ideas, either with yourself or others.

Exercise: Memory Capture

We start this section with an exercise. What is the difference between an experience and experiencing something?

> *An experience is not something that can be filed away in a notebook or captured on film and pasted into an album. Experiencing is the feeling of wonder itself, the thrill of communion, the gentle touch of our connectedness with all that surrounds us. Osho*

This exercise is designed to help support you in becoming more present when you are experiencing good, happy, or joyful moments. The idea is to be more present in the moment by experiencing it on multiple levels. Research has indicated that being more present, particularly when using mindful practices, may positively influence memory absorption. Through consciously engaging with the moment by accessing it through multiple senses, and on this occasion not taking a photograph or trying to get the best selfie, we can potentially increase our awareness, and our brain may be able to absorb and store it more vividly. In doing this you may consciously make it a part of who you are, and having stored the moment in deeper clarity and connected at the time to the positive feelings, it could become easier to access this positive memory and sensations in later, darker or more difficult moments.

We begin by practicing with an old memory, and then import the technique into the next good moment that we have. It does not need to be a big event or moment. It can be as simple as the cashier smiling at you kindly, enjoying a soothing cup of tea or completing a task.

Choose a recent or past memory that you recall feeling good, then answer the following:

1. What was happening at that moment?
2. Were you alone or were others there?
3. Which senses were activated (sight, smell, touch, taste, sound)?
4. What was the feeling in your body? Did it make you feel light, energized, relaxed, safe? Was this feeling all over or just in one place? Did you feel it elsewhere like your heart, or in your smile?
5. What did you contribute to making this moment occur or were you just a witness to it?
6. What thoughts did you have about yourself? I am being liked, recognized, heard, cared for, loved, etc.
7. What can you take from this memory to help support you in tougher times?

1. Setting the Mind

"Those who cannot change their minds cannot change anything."

George Bernard Shaw

Thus far, we have established that when we wish to change our behaviour or emotions, our ability to do so may be negatively impacted by the conditioning that we have been exposed to across our life and reinforced by our environments and experiences. Even though we attempt to address and change what we are doing, we could return to previous unhelpful or even harmful behaviours if we are not also changing the beliefs we carry about ourselves. Fortunately, our brain is not the fixed, rigid, immovable object we might think it is. Neuroplasticity is the concept that what you do and think can change the structure of your brain. This theory looks at the ways in which the brain changes in response to what we do, think, and experience in both our internal world (our minds) and our external world (the people and physical world around us). The idea is that we can possibly change or affect our experiences through changing how we think. That our abilities can change throughout our lifetime (not just as young children). Neuroplasticity tells us that the brain is not static or hardwired, but instead is plastic, flexible, and therefore changeable. In short, this means we could potentially train our brains to change.

1. Setting the Mind

Flexible Brains

We know from neuroplasticity research that the brain rewires itself by blocking neural pathways, unmasking alternative pathways, or sprouting new ones. This can occur through repetition or conscious effort, and happens naturally and spontaneously. Brain mapping and wiring can be impaired by trauma and chronic stress, be it physical, emotional, mental or even collective consciousness stress. If collective consciousness is not a term you are familiar with, it was first introduced by French sociologist Émile Durkheim. It is the unification of shared beliefs, ideas, and moral attitudes that connect a society. In the collective consciousness it is not only the positives that are shared, but also stressors, and the experience of distress can be felt on the individual level. The Covid-19 pandemic is a good example of collective consciousness having a negative impact, where most people experienced severe stress, even those who were not directly affected by the illness itself. Research suggests that generational stress can be passed down through the neural pathways. This phenomenon has been particularly observed in indigenous races that have been colonised in recent history. This makes it even more relevant that we find ways to heal and safeguard our future generations.

We previously believed our brains became set at a certain age, and that we could not change them. Instead of being able to adopt a mindset that would be appropriate to our situation and could be changed according to needs, we believed we had a mind that was unalterable, a set mind. Neuroplasticity has challenged this, and epigenetics has now shown us that thinking can turn on gene expression and form new connections between brain cells. Whilst the process is not quite as simple as this very basic explanation, without diving deeper into the technicalities of the science, essentially, what this tells us is that thoughts and beliefs can potentially change our brain structure, consequently impacting our health and wellbeing.

A set mind is not adaptable, and neither is it sustainable. Those with a set mind do not believe they can change, or at times, do not even desire to change or alter themselves in accordance with what might work better for them or others. A set mind is the antithesis to what Adaptable Sustainable Psychology (ASP) hopes to achieve. Being inflexible might not always well as a dynamic as it can automatically exclude co-operation and collaboration. When the mind is set, there is no chance for growth or betterment. A set mind may start with something like a "it is what it is" attitude graduating and becoming a "why make waves" before moving onto "I can't be bothered." It could be the place where motivation and volition go to die. Reframing our perspective and creating a mindset that is founded on flexibility, adaptability, and sustainability is possibly going to serve us much more supportively.

A mindset is a way of being that supports you in growing and changing beliefs and altering values as you evolve. This way of being may facilitate you in moving from avoiding fear to managing fear, and might give you access to ways that could support self-belief and cultivate faith that you can cope with whatever comes your way. It is a can-do attitude, not a can't-be-bothered attitude. It could help you recall those moments you have overcome and survived experiences so that you could approach future issues with a mindset of "I have done it before, I will do it again" or reliving better times and having hope of finding them again. In a mindset mode, you may find it easier to access and action your psychodiversity—your collection of

1. Setting the Mind

coping tools, ways of being, and skills used to cope with life—to examine multiple solutions and select the one that suits the circumstances. It places you more in the position of being the solution-focused storyteller, not the problem-focused storyteller. The solution-focused storyteller is one who explains what the issues are but also tells you what they are doing to manage or change them. A problem-focused storyteller only tells you what is wrong. Maybe take some time to reflect whether you have a growth mindset or a set mind. Are you running old tapes in your head using a negative narrative that puts you down rather than uplifts you? Do you think change is out of your reach? Do you focus on only the problems, or do you seek solutions as well? Neuroplasticity tells us that even if we have developed a set or fixed mind, we can change this. By switching to see our potential, we could create a better experience for ourselves in the moment, and support our wellness when problems come along later.

 The therapeutic techniques and reflective skills explored in this book are intended to support gradual, compassionate self-awareness and emotional growth. These strategies may assist you in shifting from a set mind to a mindset, centred on being more flexible, and seeking responsive ways of approaching life's challenges. Rather than relying solely on willpower, you may find that these approaches offer sustainable pathways for change that align with your values and needs. By learning some of the foundational concepts behind these methods—such as how the brain develops in response to experiences and social influences—you may begin to create a personal framework that supports emotional wellbeing. This process can invite you to gently reconsider habits that may no longer serve you and explore options that contribute to a more balanced and fulfilling way of living.

If you're looking for a quick fix or instant solution, this approach may not meet that expectation. Developing new ways of thinking and responding, sometimes called brain retraining, is typically a gradual process. It can feel repetitive at times, especially in a world filled with distractions and fast-paced demands on your attention. Like any skill, these techniques often require consistent practice and personal commitment across different aspects of life, be it mental, emotional, or physical, and for some spiritual. Making a decision to change is one part of the journey, but applying that change in daily life can take time and effort. With ongoing engagement, however, many people find that new habits can become more intuitive and easier to apply. Some individuals notice benefits from reflective practices within a few weeks, particularly when approached with regularity and intention. Over time, these tools may begin to feel more natural and integrated into everyday routines. This book offers resources that may support you in working towards a more balanced and personally meaningful life, one that reflects who you are and how you wish to move through the world. Cultivating a mindset that you choose to live from, not one adversely or negatively influenced by others.

Exercise: Grounding-Kindness Meditation

Stilling and quieting the mind to find compassion for yourself and others is a core skill in your psychodiverse toolbox. Once you feel grounded in an attitude of compassion and kindness you may find it easier to navigate more comfortably into areas of your life that you wish to change. It is in this compassionate and kind state that you might hear what your mind is up to without leaping to negative judgments that could shutdown the whole process. It could give you access to what your inner self is saying about you, cueing you into any negative beliefs that you may then choose to target if they are causing you psychological or emotional discomfort or blocking change.

One of the easiest and fastest ways to connect into yourself and focus your mind is by using your breath. Your breath is under your control, even if at times it feels like it is not (unless you have a respiratory condition). We share many different breathing techniques in this book, so you can see which ones, if any, suit you the best. After you have found ones that work for you, you can start to regularly practice them every day, even if it is for just a few minutes, maybe you can do them as you drift off to sleep, when you are driving, scrolling on your phone, getting dressed, or even on the toilet. There are so many little windows in your day where you might be able to integrate these simple exercises into your daily life.

Engaging in regular breathwork practice may support your body and mind in developing a helpful association between the technique and a sense of calm. Over time, and with consistent use, some people find that their ability to access this calming response becomes more intuitive during moments of mild to moderate stress.

While breathwork can be a valuable resource for emotional regulation, it may not be effective or appropriate in every situation, particularly in times of acute distress or when more intensive support is needed. In such cases, different strategies or professional support may be more suitable. This exercise is offered as a proactive, everyday tool to help you build emotional awareness and potentially respond to stress with greater ease. Throughout the Adaptable Sustainable Psychology collection, you'll encounter other techniques that may work better for you when managing more intense emotional experiences.

This exercise is a take on an ancient Buddhist practice that cultivates goodwill and universal friendliness toward oneself and others.

- Find a comfortable position, either sitting or lying down.
- If you feel comfortable and it is safe (i.e. you are not driving or operating machinery), close your eyes or hold a soft gaze.
- Maybe you place a hand gently on your body as a gesture of self-comfort.
- As you inhale, say quietly in your mind "in for me."
- As you exhale, say "out for others," and repeat.
- Repeat for 1 minute or longer if you can and repeat throughout the day.

1. Setting the Mind

Exercise: Train Your Brain to Change

Now that your mind is a touch quieter and hopefully more receptive to hearing that inner voice, we can look at the next step of the program to train your brain to change. To affirm is to declare positively or firmly. It is to maintain something to be true. Affirmations can be a way of telling your brain that something is already in existence. They bring change into the present, not transferring it to the future. For example, instead of, "I will stop smoking," you affirm, "I am stopping smoking." With this, you are stating you are currently stopping smoking (even if you are not), rather than waiting for a future that can never arrive as the future does not technically exist. There is only now.

Creating a personal affirmation may offer a supportive way to reinforce new, more helpful ways of thinking. Affirmations can be used as a gentle reminder of the values or beliefs you wish to strengthen. They may assist you in exploring and reframing thoughts that contribute to distress or unhelpful behavioural patterns. For instance, if you have noticed a tendency to avoid being alone due to discomfort or fear, you might choose to work with an affirmation such as: "I am learning to enjoy my own company, and I trust myself to navigate life's challenges. I value relationships that are healthy and supportive." This approach is not a substitute for therapeutic support but can be a useful part of your personal reflection and self-development.

It can be a challenge to find the underlying belief behind a negative self-statement or think of a positive counter to it. At the end of this book, you will find a series of alternative self-talk tables to help you find inspiration to create positive self-statements. Sometimes, when you have spent years thinking only difficult or dark thoughts about yourself, coming up with a positive statement can be really hard. If you struggle to work out some affirmations to counter your negative self-talk and harmful beliefs, look through the tables for ideas, and then put these statements into your own language to feel and sound like your words (not mine).

If you find this exercise brings up difficult emotions, please pause and consider seeking support from a therapist or mental health professional.

Brain Retraining Step 1:

→ Go back and review the initial identity exercises from Book 1. If you haven't completed these, instead write a list of the common negative statements you make about yourself—whether in your own mind or to others—including recurring self-criticisms, negative feedback that you ruminate on, or thoughts that cast yourself in a bad light. Look at your negative "I" statements (such as I can't cope with stress; or I am ugly; I avoid my feelings by drinking) and write a list of anything that is not helping you or is making you feel uncomfortable emotions. Compassionately, listen to that inner voice and see what you are telling yourself that is not helping.

→ Next, look for what the underlying beliefs or values might be, (there could be several) and finally, write a positive affirmation as a counter statement. An example of the process is given here in a table format to help guide you. If you struggle to identify the underlying beliefs or values of your negative self-statements, talk to people you trust or a therapist to help work out which beliefs or values your negative self-statements relate to. You may, invariably, find most relate back eventually to a feeling of not being good enough.

Negative statement about yourself	Underlying beliefs or values	Potential positive affirmation
I am always making mistakes	This could connect to believing you must do everything to an extremely high standard. Or you value doing things perfectly all the time. It could relate to fearing disapproval from others and believing you aren't worth much. Or a deep feeling of not being good enough and you can only see the things you do wrong. You might doubt your ability to change or have had others make you doubt this.	I have done some good things and can always learn how to improve. I value my efforts always. It's ok to make mistakes, we all do. I accept myself even if I make mistakes. I am more than my mistakes; I am capable of change. I can be kinder to myself when I make mistakes and encourage and support myself. I trust myself to learn and grow. I can do this. I'm doing OK.

1. Setting the Mind

I feel ugly	Are you comparing yourself to others or an ideal of how you should look, and because you are different you don't feel good enough? Have other people told you bad things about yourself and you believe them? Do you have a value that equates how you look with your self-worth, where did this come from? You? The media? Others? Is this value only applicable to yourself, can others not look perfect and still be OK and yet, you can't?	Everyone is completely unique and it's ok to look different. I can accept myself as I am and see my individual beauty. I can be kinder about my looks and appreciate that I have many other things that make me attractive as well as my appearance. I accept how other people look and see their good qualities, I can do the same for myself. I value and respect others and see the whole person, I can do that for me too. I am ok to be me.

Brain Retraining Step 2:

Once you have your affirmations, use the following steps every day for at least 30 days to help them start to take root within your brain and continue for as long as you can. Remember, it may take 12 months or even longer for new beliefs to be installed, developing neural pathways simply takes time and repetition, there are no shortcuts.

1. Repeat them out loud at least 10 times a day.
2. Write them out once a day.
3. Put them on posters around the house. Place them in areas you will see often (the fridge, the back of the bathroom door, the mirror or the first place you look when you wake up).
4. Make one affirmation a day out of playdoh or modelling clay, make the letters of each word and spell the whole affirmation out. (This can take ages if your affirmation is long so maybe do it whilst watching the television or chatting with someone.)
5. Vocally or visually record them on your phone and listen to them.
6. If you have a mobile phone, tablet or computer make affirmations into photos by writing key words on a plain or neutral background, then set this as your lock screen so that you see the keywords to prompt you back to your affirmation every time you open your device.

→ Maybe use the same part of every day for your affirmations so they become more habitual and part of your regular routine. This way you might not find it as hard to achieve the goal of daily repetition.

→ Look for times in your day where there is already a habitual task that also could include the affirmations. For example, you could say the affirmations out loud or listen to them as you shower or get dressed, when exercising, walking the dog, doing the shopping, during a meal or when commuting.

1. Setting the Mind

- → If you're shy, you can pull the posters down when you have visitors, though keeping them up may give you a chance to talk about them and share with others, helping with further forms of repetition and positive reinforcement. It may even inspire others to do the same.

- → We can get externally surrounded by fear-based narratives and internally immersed in negative narratives, these affirmations are ways you might fill your world with the more positive and supportive kinds of self-reflection and self-talk to aid in counteracting negative dynamics.

Other Suggestions:

Another technique you could consider accessing is The Emotional Freedom Technique (EFT), created by Gary Craig, it is a complementary therapy aid described as a form of psychological acupressure that uses light tapping to stimulate traditional Chinese acupuncture points. Tapping on the designated points on the face and body is combined with verbalising an identified problem, followed by a general affirmation phrase. It is another method to potentially help you change unhelpful ways of thinking and behaving that are not serving you. EFT is safe, easy to apply, and is non-invasive. Using EFT in combination with other neuroplasticity techniques may help solidify and accelerate behavioural changes. You can find EFT practitioners who are trained in providing this therapeutic technique or there are many books that may support you in developing your own practice.

Exercise: The Memory Palace

One of psychiatrist Carl Jung's well-known metaphors was to associate the structure and features of a house with aspects of the human personality and psyche. He viewed the house as a symbolic representation of the individual's inner world, with different parts of the house corresponding to different aspects of the self. The method of loci (MOL), sometimes referred to as the Memory palace, is a mnemonic device that relies on spatial relationships between locations on a familiar route, or rooms in a familiar building, to organise and recall information. By combining Jung's metaphor with this memory technique, you may be able to support the recall of your more helpful ways of thinking and responding. Over time, this practice could potentially influence the beliefs you hold about yourself and how you care for yourself in challenging moments.

Start by selecting a building or route that you're familiar with, one that does not carry any traumatic or significantly negative associations. It doesn't necessarily need to be a real building. It could be an imagined place you've envisioned for years, a dream house or a peaceful beach, or a calming forest. If buildings bring distress, choose a natural environment that feels emotionally neutral and safe. What matters most is that you can clearly connect with or visualise the place, as if you could mentally walk through it.

1. Setting the Mind

Now, you can use this palace to build associations with what you'd like to learn—whether it's a series of affirmations, a more compassionate way of supporting yourself, or a new emotional self-care habit. You can use rooms or locations that symbolise or correlate with the person you are aiming to become or the behaviours you seek to adopt as habits, aim to include unusual or out-of-place objects or characters. This novelty can improve recall by standing out vividly against a familiar background. Once you have designed your memory palace it can be used repeatedly for memorisation.

It may take some time to design and internalise your memory palace, but the goal is that, in the long term, it might support you in adopting more adaptive self-care practices or beliefs. Let yourself be creative, have fun and make the experience meaningful.

Example to Help Get You Started:

- At the entrance to your chosen location, whether it's a forest trail, a beach, or the front gate of your dream house, imagine a welcome mat or sign. Picture a cheerful frog, hedgehog, or any character that makes you smile, holding a sign that reads: *"Welcome. Be gentle with yourself."*

- As you enter the hallway, or pass an internet café on the beach, or a video booth in the forest, you receive a video call. Perhaps it's from a penguin, Kermit the Frog, or another delightfully unexpected character. The caller tells you, in a kind and clear tone, to stop saying negative or unkind things to yourself.

- Next, move to a space symbolising nourishment—a kitchen, a food stall, or a cosy café nestled in the trees. Here, maybe Big Bird is cooking for you, or a giraffe is preparing a snack. These comforting characters gently remind you to offer yourself kindness and support when life feels difficult.

- In the office or study, there's a quirky bin in the shape of a monkey, or maybe a colourful, out-of-place sheep. You write down a self-critical belief like "I'm a failure," "I'm not worthy," or "I can't change." You scrunch the paper, toss it into the bin, and watch the monkey do a little dance or hear a sheep make a cheerful *baa* in celebration of your effort to let go of that belief.

- In the lounge, or around a clearing in the forest or a beachside seating area, you sit in an oversized polka-dot armchair, hugging the softest cushion you can imagine. The cushion bears a simple but powerful message: *"I can cope. I can come through this."*

- In the bathroom mirror, you see your hair transformed into your favourite bold colour. On the mirror are the words: *"I am doing okay."*

- Finally, the bedroom—your most personal, private space. Here, picture a version of yourself feeling truly enough. Perhaps you're dressed in the most joyful, vibrant outfit you can imagine, and you feel fabulous in it. Or maybe there's a large photograph of you, looking peaceful and content. Or you sit on the most comfortable bed ever and hold something deeply meaningful: a pet, jewellery, car keys, anything symbolic. On the wall, in bold letters, it says: *"I'm glad I'm me."*

1. Setting the Mind

Once your memory palace is built, it can be used repeatedly for memorization. Regular practice helps make the palace more efficient and the recall process more natural.

1. Maybe you read it many times throughout the day.
2. Or spend time visualising yourself walking through it again, and again and again.
3. Record yourself describing your memory palace and listen to it as often as possible.
4. If you need to recall the information to support yourself in a tough moment or after you have witnessed yourself being self-critical, return to mentally walking through your memory palace, observing the images you placed in each area. The images should trigger the associated information, allowing you to recall what you need in that difficult moment.

If you need to add in anything new to your memory palace you can simply walk into another room or area and add relevant images, associating the images with the information you wish to retain. You can also reuse the same palace for entirely different information or even add new details or perspectives to it as needed.

Pause — Reflect — Landscape

We are working on developing our own Adaptable Sustainable Psychology, so we may learn how to help ourselves feel better, treat ourselves better and treat others better. At the end of each section, we want to reinforce and integrate any new knowledge. Reflecting on the material in relation to ourselves and our life can help with this, and, where relevant, show us where we may adjust accordingly.

1. Pause - Take a moment to sit with what you have just learned and consider it.

- Neuroplasticity and epigenetics show us that we can potentially change the structure of our brains through thinking.
- The brain can be rewired by blocking or overriding unhelpful pathways and making new ones through spontaneous events and repetition.
- Trauma, chronic stress, collective consciousness stress and intergenerational trauma can impact how our brain is structured and functions and may affect our self-belief.
- A set mind may not allow for adaptation and could become unsustainable and then may limit our potential.

1. Setting the Mind

- A mindset is an attitude or way of being that encourages, embraces and supports growth and change.
- Retraining our brains to develop a positive, healthy and affirming mindset may take time and a lot of repetition, both patience and commitment can help with this.
- There are brain retraining techniques that can help support us in gradually and compassionately transforming unhelpful or harmful beliefs.

2. Reflect - Answer the following questions:

- Do you think you have a limiting set mind or have a mindset that is open to and supportive of growing and changing?
- Have you identified some beliefs about yourself that are not necessarily promoting and supporting your confidence, your wellbeing or your ability to feel good enough?
- Are there aspects of your personality or history that might make long-term repetitive training a challenge for you?

3. Landscape - Step back from the details and see how this new information fits in with the bigger picture of your life. Consider your history, what is going on for you now, who and what is in your life, and the future you want for yourself.

→ When you look back over your life, and using the 3 identity maps (on yourself, your parent/caregivers and your culture/society) that you have completed from book 1 or your list of negative thoughts, what do you think might have influenced how you think about the process of change itself, and can you identify anything that may affect your ability to maintain a program to change?

→ What kind of mindset could work well for you, the relationships you have and the goals or dreams you are working towards? What beliefs about yourself might you need to change or alter to create this kind of mindset?

→ Have you tried using brain retraining techniques previously? Were they useful? If they were not supportive, can identify what stopped them from being more effective in supporting change? Do you have any insights or ideas that could mitigate or manage blocks to maintaining repetitive techniques that support change?

2. Being Human is Not Easy

In this section you will be learning about:

- → How being human isn't simple, and trying to force it to be is not effective or helpful.
- → Why understanding complexity is useful when we want to create change.
- → How we might be using unhelpful coping tools.
- → Why implicit and confirmation biases feed our fears and do not permit growth.
- → How to use 'witness mode' to reduce stress and foster understanding, growth, and change.

You will need:

- ✓ To be ready to work with your reality, and to do work that might be complex, foregoing simplicity.
- ✓ Quiet time to practice some breathwork.
- ✓ Awareness that trying an exercise only once is not going to create a lasting habit.
- ✓ Determination to develop an ongoing daily practice with repetitive exercises.
- ✓ Pen and paper to make notes on insights that arise.
- ✓ To be open to discussing your reactions, feelings, and ideas, either with yourself or others.

2. Being Human is Not Easy

"I never lose, I either win or learn."

Nelson Mandela

If exploring what it means to be human can contribute to supporting change, making improvements in health, wellbeing, and resilience, then reflecting on the many factors that influence our behaviour, whether consciously or unconsciously, may be a helpful starting point. Developing a broader perspective on who we are, what has shaped us, and how internal and external influences may affect us can support greater self-awareness and personal insight. When we gain a clearer understanding of our patterns and preferences, it may become easier to strengthen our core sense of self and respond with more flexibility during times of stress or uncertainty, enhancing and supporting any processes of change we are undertaking.

The human experience is inherently complex, and each of us navigates life without a predetermined map, making self-reflection a valuable process for meaningful growth. Accepting complexity could be beneficial when seeking to support changes within yourself. The minute you want it to be simple; you may naturally look for the quick fix. In a modern world where technology is evolving faster than we are, where instantaneous results are beginning to be expected continuously, where perfection is seemingly constantly attained, we can run the risk of becoming unreasonable and demanding of ourselves. Looking for a simple change when there might be layers and levels that may also need to be explored and worked on could leave us disappointed and disheartened. We can be complex; change can be complex. Working with complexity with a positive and accepting mindset may well help to increase your chances of success.

Refusing the complex for the simple can stem from not wanting to do the work. The avoidance of any perceived hard work may prevent us from reaching our goals, because typically, we are going to have do the work if we are going to achieve worthwhile things. Wanting simple fixes can be a kind of avoidance or a form of denial; both of which may lead to a loss of our personal resources, like time and energy. At times, it is likely to be more effective to get into the glorious, detailed complexity of it all from the start. Given how much information we are exposed to daily (remember 74 gigabytes), it is no small wonder we want things to be simpler. We become overwhelmed more quickly with the increasingly large rush of information demanding to be processed. We instinctually do not want to add to this cognitive or emotional load. Hence, we develop simplicity-seeking behaviours that we all practice at times. This is something everyone does. It's a natural part of being human, we try to conserve energy where we can, so don't feel bad or judge it negatively.

But when it comes to managing ourselves and caring for how we set our minds up, this is not an area to skimp on or skip over. Social media is a good example of the seemingly simple potentially being annoyingly complex. Social media, in many ways, portrays itself as a simple tool to access and connect with friends. Yet, ironically, surfing social media absorbs

2. Being Human is Not Easy

a huge amount of our time and emotional energy. Taking real-time opportunities to be with people away. It is not uncommon to see couples or groups of people spending time together, all sitting and looking at their devices, not actually engaging with one another. Furthermore, thanks to the subtle triggering and activating effects of reading about everyone's lives or scrolling past the numerous adverts to get to something relevant, we are often being drained without necessarily realising it. Taking our focus and energy resources. What seems simple becomes complex. Working your way through so many opinions, perfect photos, or people's frustrations is not a simple way to connect with others or ease your mind and spend your time. Exposure to all these emotions could confuse your own feelings, and that simplicity you're seeking is replaced by another layer of complexity in an already overburdened mind. Using socially media mindfully, with an awareness of how it can affect you, may help with this.

When seeking an attitude of simplicity with one area of life, there is a chance we might generalise this brand of thinking to every other area. Humans are always trying to unconsciously preserve energy. Thus, if there is a short cut, we might take it. If we can opt out, we possibly will. If we can keep repeating behaviours that use less energy output rather than changing behaviours that require a higher energy output, we could do so to conserve energy. Energy is equal to survival. We save it where we can. Remember, this is a human thing, not a you thing. There's no need to beat yourself up about it, but it is helpful to be aware of it and manage it.

One danger of simplification is that we set ourselves up with such a narrow bandwidth of thinking that we can become rooted or stuck in unhelpful patterns of behaviour and this may prevent us from being able to make changes. For instance, we can have a series of bad relationships, and then unconsciously make a simple assumption that all men, or all women are going to be out to hurt us. This kind of limiting thinking could lead us to judging others unfairly, feeling overwhelmingly afraid or reduce our opportunities to be able to openly accept the possibility of positive interactions. We might see this limited style of thinking also play out in cultural stereotyping. For example, people could simply assume they are seeing a man when going to see a new doctor, or that any nurse they meet will be female. The term for this is called unconscious bias. We all use this tool, so don't judge yourself harshly. It happens without conscious engagement, it is an automatic behaviour that can influence our decisions, judgments, and behaviour without us wanting it to. By becoming aware of it we may be able to manage any possible negative impacts it could have on us.

As we touched on in Book 1, humans typically like to feel they belong. They need a sense of being a part of something, whether it is big or small. This means, if you have a narrow way of looking at your self-development, then you are likely to go and seek out those who reinforce and support this, rather than challenge it. We can unconsciously seek out opportunities to reinforce our behaviour and maintain where we are, looking for ways to validate what we believe through so-called 'evidence.' This is called confirmation bias. We find someone outside of ourselves who shares our belief. Therefore, it must be true, and no complex or hard work is required to change. The original belief could then be laid in deeper and become harder to challenge or change. Diversity becomes the enemy. This is definitely not a psychodiverse way to live.

2. Being Human is Not Easy

When unconscious bias and confirmation bias become companions, we could have a problem. Imagine going to a friend you know who shares your views on things, and asking them for their advice. Because you are like minded, they confirm what you were already telling yourself, making the advice possibly redundant. Imagine picking out small sections of someone's complaint to make yourself the victim rather than seeing things from the other person's side or being accountable for your part in the situation. Imagine only choosing select parts of what a therapist has said to you, or that you have read in a self-help book, and ignoring the rest to suit your current narrative, so you have less work to do. With these two biases collaborating, you can keep replaying the same small segment of the story that works for you, miss the bigger picture, and not enter into the complexity that might be required for change to occur. This is not to say that seeking out similar opinions from others is always bad. Sometimes, we are right to check in and validate appropriate thoughts and beliefs with those we are aligned with. But we may need to question things from time to time and realise that we can unconsciously and automatically avoid potentially different perspectives, instead of looking for them. You may need to ask yourself:

- Am I absolutely correct in my thinking?
- Where has this thinking come from, could it be an unhelpful, overly simple or an unfair stereotype?
- Am I just checking in with sources that might back me up because it's easier than risking having to change?
- Do I fear there is more complexity here because of trauma or past experiences that are very painful to look at?

By gently and compassionately questioning yourself, without adding judgment to your responses, you might be able to see where you could be avoiding complexity in favour of simplicity and assess if this is going to serve you both now and possibly in the future, or if you might need to address the deeper and bigger issues or seek professional help in doing so.

Being in a state of metacognition means you are thinking about your way of thinking, checking if it is helpful, not just now but in the long-term as well. For example, your drinking buddy may agree to go to the pub with you, after you told them it has been a hard day. But if you then go on to have many more drinks and repeat this every night, this might not be serving your liver long-term. As a coping mechanism for stress, it probably isn't great and seeking out the friend you know also drinks too much alcohol is not going to help the situation either. These two types of bias may become the toxic twins that stop you from seeing what you are doing to yourself, things that are not helping you to live a better life or connect well with others. These biases can block change and reduce our psychodiversity and then adaptation may not be possible.

Being able to face difficult things about ourselves can be supported through our courage.

Courage can help support us when coming to terms with who we are and what needs working on. Courage can help us in really taking in another point of view, to ask questions of ourselves, and to pay attention to areas of being human that might trip us up. Finding pathways to our personal courage may help us in this process of change. From this place of courage and clarity, we may identify whether we are simplicity seeking or

2. Being Human is Not Easy

complexity avoidant, and then we can then shift our thinking, to our benefit and to the benefit of others.

Whilst we might be courageous, we can still be fearful, and fear may lie beneath some of our biases, and can be potentially harmful when it does. We may use confirmation bias because we fear change, or we are afraid that we might be in the wrong, or that we might need to take accountability for things we have done previously and this scares us in case of terrible repercussions, especially if we have had traumatic experiences of being unfairly or over-harshly punished. We can also generate biases based on fears of losing resources, and this may be where the difficulty comes in.

A useful acronym of FEAR is False Evidence Appearing Real. What this means is that we can take a part of the truth, expand it into a much bigger story and then create a whole terrible story with a series of consequences that do not necessarily have anything to do with the current reality. Racism is a good example of how fear can drive our biases. We could be told by the news that an influx of immigrants seeking public housing are causing a crisis, and we then may create an inaccurate stereotype that all immigrants are taking our resources (this is an unconscious bias). Our fear of losing these resources and there not being enough could blind us from seeing the immigrants who come into the country and earn their living, paying their own way in the private housing sector from working hard. We share this biased perspective with others, who also fear immigrants, and because if others believe it to be true then it must be, our perspective is confirmed and allows us to think that we were right to be afraid (confirmation bias). The fear that sits beneath the biases does not allow us to see other facts and hear evidence that could contradict this racist view.

The combination of fear and bias can fight to keep us oblivious to other points of view, always finding fault with contrary perspectives. Breaking through this kind of fear and bias could be very challenging.

We know that **diversity can enhance and improve our lives**. When we embrace learning about other people's thoughts, ideas, perspectives or ways of living, we have chances to increase our own awareness and empathy. When our minds remain fluid, flexible, and open, the voice of the past and limitation may not dominate the present as significantly, and we could improve our chances to actively learn and have new or different experiences of something that might have previously been harmful, painful or difficult. It does not mean we end up agreeing or taking up another's ideas necessarily, but it can afford us an opportunity to better understand one another from a place of kindness and compassion. We can still retain our independence, and we might upgrade to interdependence, where we connect and co-operate to allow one another's views to co-exist respectfully. Learning to re-record those unhelpful tapes in our mind that stop us from believing we can change, or that we are enough might then allow us to actively encourage diversity, and this could open our mindset to be able to embrace opportunities for personal and collective growth. Instead of opting for the simple we might experience and benefit from the complex.

Unconscious bias and confirmation bias can block our capacity to change until we allow ourselves shift into witness mode, where balanced, conscious observation can more likely occur. **Witness mode** is a calm, nonjudgmental, and open mindset that focuses on taking in a broad range of information from all points of view. Learning how to switch into witness mode can help break down these biases and stop them boxing us in the corner of a set mind and hindering change. When we witness something, we do not judge, we can manage the influence of the past to recognise it might not be the same situation here in the present as it was before, and we may then take in information and assess it more fairly and accurately from a broader perspective. This method may prevent fear and bias from escalating, and could help alleviate our stress and support us towards appropriate and sustainable changes. Instead of living in a future of absolutes that might not be accurate, we can accept possibility and opportunity, and this may well be a much nicer space to experience life from.

Exercise: Witnessing Breathing

This centering breathwork may assist you in learning how to remain calm and witness yourself, others or your environment. When you start the practice of the witnessing your breath, you may then be able to apply witnessing techniques to your thoughts, your behaviours, and to the world around you, giving you access to the pause button to assess a broader perspective, rather than potentially focusing on fear or other biases that may not support your wellbeing, create healthy connections or capacity to change.

Remember, the more you practice these daily habits, the easier it may become for your brain to develop the ability to access them to help you in difficult moments and can help your body to become familiar with what this calm and observant space feels like. You can find a recording of this exercise on our website.

- Focus your attention completely on the centre of your forehead.
- Bring every thought, every scrap of awareness to the centre of your forehead, between your eyebrows.
- Breathe in and out of your nose if you can. If not, use your mouth.

2. Being Human is Not Easy

- Consciously feel your brow relax and let go whilst keeping your focus on the centre of it.
- Witness the air coming in and out of the body whilst maintaining complete focus on the centre of your forehead.
- As you breathe in, count silently from 1 to 4.
- As you breathe out, count silently from 1 to 4.
- Repeat this several times, in for 4, out for 4.
- Keep an even breath and maintaining your focus entirely on the centre of your forehead.
- If your mind wanders, don't judge yourself. Simply return to focusing on the centre of your forehead and your counting.
- Let thoughts arrive and then let them go without following them.
- Gently reorient the mind if it moves away by coming back to the counting and the centre of your forehead.
- Observe how the breath fills the body then eases away.
- Feel into the parts of your body that are softening and loosening.
- Take note of how the silence feels between the out and the in breath, how still it is.
- Be present with every part of the breath.
- Witness the gap at the end of each exhalation and remain focused on the centre of your forehead.
- Continue for as long as you can, counting in rounds of 4.

Pause — Reflect — Landscape

1. **Pause** - Take a moment to sit with what you have just learned and consider it.

    - We are complex beings, and our beliefs and behaviours are affected by many factors. The more we know ourselves, the greater the chance we have to look after ourselves.

    - Denying our complexity or avoiding the work of change may not be a good use of our resources. We may benefit from the awareness that seemingly simple activities may add more to our cognitive and emotional load.

    - We naturally preserve energy, if we are running low on personal resources, we may pull back from high energy load activities like change, and this could affect us now or in the future.

    - Unconscious bias can lead to unhelpful stereotyping that limits us and keeps us from exploring new opportunities.

    - Confirmation bias compels us to seek out others that share our values or views and this could reduce chances to be challenged and may limit opportunities for change.

- It is wise to check in our thinking and ask if we are seeking out confirmation because it seems easier than a contrary or alternate opinion. We may be supported through finding our courage to hear alternate views that might challenge us or even change us.
- Fear can create biases that blind us and put us or others at risk.
- Diversity in our thinking increases awareness and empathy, helping possibly to make a nicer internal environment for ourselves and a better experience for others.
- Witness mode can help us break free from the hold our natural biases may have on us that might otherwise limit our capacity to change and grow.

2. **Reflect** - Answer the following questions:

- Do you think you are someone who prefers simplicity or embraces complexity?
- Do you think biases might prevent you from actioning changes? Can you see where you might be using unconscious or confirmation bias in your life, is it helpful or hindering your growth?
- Have you had a strong emotional reaction to the discussion about our biases? Why do you think that is?

3. **Landscape** - Step back from the details and see how this new information fits in with the bigger picture of your life. Consider your history, what is going on for you now, who and what is in your life, and the future you want for yourself.

- ✓ Have you found some stereotyping biases present in how you think? Can you see where they come from? Do you wish to hang onto them or could it be beneficial to work on them and let them go?
- ✓ If you have particular fears that can lead you down the path of being biased, is there value in using your courage to work on them and maybe changing your beliefs to support a more encouraging perspective to manage these fears?
- ✓ If you have experienced trauma has this impacted any biases, either positively or negatively? Is this an area that you wish to work on and could benefit from seeking professional help with?

3. Emotions as Informants

In this section you will be learning about:

- → How our emotions can tell us about things we might need to change.
- → How we can develop the ability to be comfortable when our feelings are not comfortable.
- → The importance of identifying the whole array of human emotions and how to question our feelings.
- → Being a solution-focused storyteller instead of a problem-focused storyteller.
- → Using feelings such as frustration to fuel growth.

You will need:

- ✓ To be prepared to dig deeper into your feelings to see what they may have to show you about yourself and how you are living.
- ✓ Space and time to meditate.
- ✓ A simple object such as a glass to use in meditation.
- ✓ Pen and paper to make notes on any insights that arise.
- ✓ To be open to discussing your reactions, feelings, and ideas, either with yourself or others.

3. Emotions as Informants

"Change is inevitable. Growth is optional."
John Maxwell

Our emotions can be integral to our capacity to grow and thrive. They are an important aspect of being human and, when harnessed with mindful care, they can help us progress and flourish. Emotions could be viewed as informants providing us with valuable insights. They can act as an alarm or cue that something is either going right or amiss, alerting us to potential problems or danger. Generally speaking, we can categorise emotions into two types of experience. There are comfortable emotions like peace, joy, happiness, contentment, etc., that we might be more likely to experience in our awareness state. Then, there are uncomfortable emotions that may be ego generated, such as guilt, anger, frustration, grief, misery, etc. Becoming comfortable with the uncomfortable emotions can assist us in managing and coping with life and the difficult moments that can occur. But learning to be comfortable with uncomfortable emotions can be a hard skill to attain and one that may take time. Part of achieving this transformative skill comes from learning to understand what our emotions are showing us, learning to see how they can inform us as to what is working and what is not. They may be reflecting how we are thinking about something or seeing ourselves. They could relate to another person or a trauma, accident, or event. Remember, **everything shows you something.**

Whether the origin of the emotion is internal, (from our thoughts), or external, (from events or other people), emotions have the power to reveal our beliefs and values relating to that experience. Whilst our beliefs and values can be influenced, ultimately, they are under our control, meaning if a belief or value surfaces that we do not like or does not serve us well, we can change it, and this may then provide an opportunity for our feelings to evolve and become more manageable. When choosing your thoughts, you provide yourself with the ability to change how you are seeing either yourself or the circumstance you are in and therefore, potentially change your emotional experience of it. We must be careful not to oversimplify this. If someone attacks you or you have a traumatic experience, changing your thoughts is not going to change the reality of being hurt, disturbed, and distressed. But choosing how you think about yourself and the event may help you grow out of that experience and move forward.

Experiencing and processing emotions can be as equally valuable as understanding them, especially when they may become obstacles to us growing and changing. By analysing and interpreting our emotions, we may create and support their transformation, but there may be times we can benefit from feeling our feelings. Ignoring emotions could be ineffectual. They can still surface, even if we try to suppress or ignore them, whether that happens sooner or later. Emotions may show up as behaviour, physical illness, mental illness, fatigue or chronic pain. Emotions can show up in how we operate in our relationships. We may be more irritable, angry or withdrawn, or the emotional experience can front as a lack of

3. Emotions as Informants

self-confidence. Overwhelming emotions can block or prevent change altogether if not understood, supported and managed.

Being present in your emotion and responding to it by feeling it can be a good starting place. When you are present you can assign the emotion to the relevant situation and respond to that emotional experience. If you are reacting to the feeling without engaging with it, then you risk, perhaps unconsciously, bringing past feelings into the present that could confuse the issue, adding excess emotion that might not be helpful and may lead you to feeling overwhelmed. By being present, you are dealing with the situation you are in. You can actively manage any past similar emotional experiences, be aware of possible future fears, or identify behaviours that are not helpful or relevant. When you are present, you can truly feel this feeling, which may be difficult and challenging. But when you allow yourself to feel your uncomfortable emotions, you may find that they don't last as long. Suppressing them, avoiding them, denying them, is generally unhelpful, they may have to be dealt with at some point and letting them fester is unlikely to be a sensible option. It can be incredibly hard to sit with uncomfortable feelings, there are good reasons we avoid doing it, but learning to find comfort in knowing they pass, that you can learn from them and you can influence and affect your own life through how you think, what you believe, and the actions you choose to take, can help you get through those difficult moments.

It can be annoying when you are in the depths and intensity of strong emotions and someone says, "this too will pass", or "you'll get over it". It could be annoying for a few reasons. Maybe, deep down, you know this to be true—or perhaps you also sense that it's not quite an absolute truth. Remember, an absolute truth is something that is always true in every circumstance, whereas a relative truth depends on your experience, knowledge, or certain conditions being met. That's why some feelings about particular situations may return—like missing a loved one, for example. What we might be better to acknowledge when hearing the phrases that can irritate us or feel unhelpful is that it is ok to surrender into the moment and support ourselves in gradually releasing the feeling in our own space and time, and to consider that the intensity can pass, the feeling of not being in control can pass and to remember that other things can occur to create easier and more pleasant emotional experiences in between these difficult moments. It's not easy to accept things can pass or believe they can change when your feelings are so big, so intense and so overwhelming, but change comes, one way or another, and you can influence how you feel about it with compassion, care and possibly some professional support along the way.

Being present and feeling the initial emotion may help you to identify not just the surface or immediate feeling, but any other relevant emotions that might be underneath that first layer. Becoming more acquainted with the nuances of emotion and the different types of feelings we can experience can help us in identifying our own feelings. Sometimes our emotional lexicon, or our understanding of all the different types of emotions might be quite narrow, finding ways to expand this, through personal research, reading up about feelings or talking to others, could be a worthwhile endeavour. For example, when receiving a negative comment, you might initially feel angry. Then, underneath this anger, you realise you feel hurt. And, underneath that hurt, you are fearful of being seen a certain way by someone who might be important

3. Emotions as Informants

to you. This information on all the emotional experiences in that one moment could help you to see that by reframing how you receive that comment, you change your feelings around it. Perhaps you can learn from it. Perhaps you realise the comment was less about you and more about the other person. Maybe you can reassure yourself that whilst the comment may hold some truth, there are other good qualities you have, and you don't necessarily need this person to see this as you know it. Thus, you can reduce the impact of what might feel like a highly and negatively personalised comment, and then not feel quite as hurt from it. Allowing you to potentially return to a stable sense of self-worth more quickly and with less suffering along the way.

When people say that they feel a certain way, they often just stop there. For example, they might say they feel anxious and nothing more. But anxiety is likely not the only emotion present. The individual might not be digging further. They may not have asked themselves questions like the following: What is it that I think could or could not happen? Is there a fear here? Is there a lack of self-belief or some self-doubt? Do I think I have no control? Is there a belief here that is driving my anxiety that might not be true? And I could change it with self-compassion, self-awareness and neural reprogramming techniques? By questioning your anxiety or any feeling you are experiencing, you may empower yourself into a more supportive and helpful line of thinking. This type of questioning of your emotions means that you can move from being a problem-focused storyteller to a **solution-focused storyteller**. In this process, you may find that anxiety or some other dominating emotion has become a coping mechanism or consequence instead of an emotional experience that could pass but somehow has got stuck. Once you have broken down the layers of the emotions you are having, it may be easier to start sorting through them and find potential solutions or opportunities for change and transformation.

Feeling our feelings and identifying all the emotional layers, developing skills to be able to become more comfortable with the uncomfortable moments, and learning to transform our emotions through our perceptions are high-level skills that may take refinement and practice. They also require a lot of self-compassion. But once you start to learn these techniques, and continue to practice them over a lifetime, it can potentially support you in those difficult moments, which may lighten the load and help ease you through them, and from this softer and lighter space change becomes more manageable and sustainable. Pain, as they say, is inevitable. But **growth is a choice.**

3. Emotions as Informants

Exercise: Observation and Witnessing Meditation

At times, it can be very hard to sit and listen to yourself, or feel your feelings, without the clutter of your mind, unhelpful thoughts, the world, or other people getting in the way, or without fearing being overwhelmed. Having a raft of different ways to tune into yourself can help build the skills and mental muscles needed to focus in what might be causing you some disturbance or distress. When you tune in directly to yourself, it is in this space you are more likely to be able to feel your feelings, identify them and work with them to move forward.

This reflective exercise is designed to help you temporarily reduce the noise of life, so you can find the stillness within and create space to gently feel into your internal emotional landscape. With regular practice, you may find it easier to access a sense of calm or focused presence. These skills often develop gradually over time. Engaging in brief, intentional pauses—even just a minute or two throughout the day—can support the development of emotional awareness and self-regulation in a way that feels manageable and sustainable.

This technique is intended to help support your capacity to witness thoughts, emotions, or bodily sensations without needing to change, judge, or react to them. Rather than engaging in active problem-solving or avoidance, the practice invites gentle awareness, acknowledging what is present and allowing it to be, while maintaining steady, calm breathing. Over time, this may assist in developing emotional regulation and a sense of inner steadiness when facing discomfort or distress.

You may start off doing this exercise in a quieter room to help you find that peaceful, inner stillness. But in time, you may find you can achieve this in a louder, noisier and more dynamic environment, thus, possibly supporting you in building the skills and strengthening that mental muscle to maintain calm in any storm, regardless of what is going on around you.

- → Sit in a comfortably seated position. Using a pre-selected inanimate object (with no writing on it or sentimental value attached to it), gaze at the object without thinking about it.
- → Witness its existence without attaching any thoughts or feelings to it.
- → If thoughts appear, acknowledge them, maybe with a silent thank you or even a nod of your head to indicate to your brain you recognise them, but you are releasing them. Do not follow them. Let them go and maintain your presence with the object and the environment.
- → Come back to the breath to aid in releasing thoughts rather than following them.
- → Inhaling to acknowledge the thought, exhaling to release the thought.

3. Emotions as Informants

→ When you feel more peaceful and centred, and you are not following your thoughts or feelings, move your gaze around the room without thinking about anything. Hear noises, feel the energy, and observe everything—being a witness without creating or listening to thoughts or feelings.

When you are completely immersed in that moment of witnessing, and it may only last for a few seconds or a minute or two, use this gentle silence to feel into the calm and centredness of the experience. As the feeling is likely only to initially last a few moments this is how you can more easily practice throughout the day, without needing to create space for a long meditation regime. One breath, one moment of stillness may make all the difference to how you feel and how you cope.

Pause — Reflect — Landscape

1. **Pause** - Take a moment to sit with what you have just learned and consider it.

- We can experience comfortable and uncomfortable emotions, and they are all useful and valid.
- Our emotions may alert us to things that might benefit from being addressed and give us insights on how to support ourselves.
- Learning how to be more comfortable with uncomfortable emotions can be transformative.
- Being present in our feeling is a good first step. This may help protect us from being overwhelmed from past emotions that might prevent us from dealing with the current feeling.
- By finding ways to feel our feelings that work for us this may aid in processing the experience and eventually letting it go.
- Feeling our feelings might at times shorten the experience of them, reduce the intensity and support our future self from becoming overwhelmed by unresolved by emotional experiences.

3. Emotions as Informants

- Looking beyond that first emotion may help us to see what else might be sitting there. This could help us resolve situations and feel freer and clearer from emotional baggage that might hamper us in the future.
- We might find it useful to learn more about different kinds of feelings we can experience, and how they show up for us, to be able to process them and move forward.
- Questioning our feelings can help us unravel the emotional layers and find solutions or opportunities that could help us feel better.
- Learning to be still, clear the clutter of the mind and feel into ourselves is a useful and supportive skill for emotional identification and emotional management.

2. **Reflect** - Answer the following questions:

- Are you someone who pays attention to your feelings or do you tend to just push them aside and get on with life?
- Have you any concerns or fears about sitting with your feelings and allowing yourself to be in the moment with them?
- How confident do you feel in recognising the different kinds of emotions we have? Do you need to learn more about emotions and ways to identify them in yourself and others?

3. **Landscape** - Step back from the details and see how this new information fits in with the bigger picture of your life. Consider your history, what is going on for you now, who and what is in your life, and the future you want for yourself.

→ Have you had experiences where past emotions impact a current situation? Does being emotionally overwhelmed affect you in maintaining changes or stop you in the process? Is this something that you would like to manage differently?

→ What are the risks of feeling your feelings? Are there opportunities that could open up from paying attention to and managing your feelings? Is this something you might need professional help with, to feel safer when exploring or feeling your emotions?

→ What questions can you ask yourself that might help you develop a greater understanding of your feelings and how you manage them? Can you put a plan in place to support any insight or ideas you have to improve your emotional management to support you in changing and growing?

4. Denial.
It's Not Just a River in Africa

In this section you will be learning about:

→ What are the four types of potentially unhelpful coping tools we can use too much?

→ What are the risks of overusing unhelpful coping tools?

→ How can we identify unhelpful coping tools?

You will need:

✓ Time to reflect and contemplate.

✓ To be open and honest with yourself about how you cope in different situations.

✓ To show yourself compassion when recognizing unhelpful patterns of behaviour.

✓ Pen and paper to carry out an exercise identifying coping mechanisms you use and how often you use them.

✓ To be open to discussing your reactions, feelings, and ideas, either with yourself or others.

4. Denial.
It's not just a river in Africa.

"Problems are not the problem; coping is the problem."
Virginia Satir

There are helpful ways to cope with our emotions or unhelpful ones that can cause us problems. A sustainable approach is one that may encourage growth, whereas an unsustainable one could cause us harm. Knowing what kinds of emotional coping mechanisms we use and how much we use them may help prevent us from adopting and maintaining unhelpful coping tools that could potentially be setting us up for future problems.

The following are four coping tools that, when used sparingly and with conscious attention, can be useful and, when unmanaged, may be harmful to us.

- Denial
- Diversion
- Distraction
- Avoidance

Whilst sometimes these tools are **potentially** useful, they are **time limited in that utility**. Excessive, long-term use is not recommended as they could become more unhelpful than helpful. Virtually everyone uses the less helpful coping mechanisms. Spare yourself any negative judgment, all of us do this at some point or another. When used consciously and carefully, and typically only in short bursts, some of these methods can be effective tools for managing difficult and/or painful situations. Unfortunately, as they tend to alleviate and temporarily displace painful and uncomfortable feelings, we are generally inclined to then use them excessively because they make us feel better. But this then may create secondary and tertiary problems that could affect our personal health, financial health, families, relationships, home, and careers.

Denial

Denial can be useful when applied with fighting spirit and determination to succeed at a task or achieve a goal. For example, research has indicated that a cancer survivor's denial that they are going to die while maintaining a fighting spirit to be healthy again has been shown to correlate with a significant increase in the chance of recovery. Denial can help you not give up until you find a way to achieve your goal, a useful way to focus energies, especially when faced with adversity or setbacks.

But denial that is used to ignore problems or not acknowledge behaviours that are either harmful to the self or others is risky. That which we deny, we can do nothing about. If someone denies that they have a drinking problem, they are obviously not going to stop drinking. A person who denies that their behaviour is harmful to another, and then combines this with a diversionary tactic to either blame the other person or a distraction tactic to focus on another unrelated issue, may provide them with the ultimate coping mechanism of avoidance. In the act of denial, the behaviour that needs changing gets lost and the damage continues. For example, you approach your partner about helping out more around the house, they snap back at you that they did the washing up last night, and they are tired from working all week. When you start to explain that you too are tired from work, and have cooked and washed up every other night that week, they interrupt, and say it wasn't so much what you asked, but the tone and the way you asked, as it reminded them of a bad previous relationship. By this time, you are focused on what you allegedly said in the wrong tone and your partner's hurt feelings from their past, rather than resolving sharing the housework more equitably. The denial from your partner about owning their fair share of the household task means the problem is not going to get addressed and resolved.

Diversion

At times, when there is little we can do about a situation, creating a diversion can help us hold steady until there is an opportunity to address the issue. By diverting energy into something we can positively influence or change, we can feel better about ourselves instead of potentially landing in helplessness with the problem we cannot do anything about at present. We might use diversion positively, through engaging in an activity that brings us comfort, confidence or joy, like gardening, a creative pursuit or hobby, planning a holiday, reliving some past happy events in our minds or talking about them, remembering someone important to us and sharing funny stories about them with other people.

However, diversion can be overused and misused. If you keep diverting yourself away from the uncomfortable matter it is not going to be resolved and could even worsen over time.

Diversion can also be one of the most subtly misused and manipulative of the unhelpful four. Diversion occurs when, for example, you wish to address an issue with someone and they propose an alternate problem, (possibly a problem originating from you and not them), and they purposely zero in on this matter as then being more important to discuss. An example of this might be, when your flatmate is not paying their share of the bills, when you go to address this with them, they tell they are being bullied at work, and that they hate their job, their boss reminds them of their abusive father and it is making them feel depressed. You get so caught up in supporting them and trying to offer them comfort that you forget all about the fact they have not been paying their fair share. Whilst you can certainly feel for them and offer some support, they still need to hold their end of the financial responsibilities and be accountable for seeking help with their depression, and maybe looking for professional support in seeking a new job. This kind of diversion can be more effective when used with someone who is naturally caring and compassionate. The diversion, in this instance, is typically laden with emotion of a prior hurt or trauma and used as leverage so that the compassionate and caring person automatically switches into caring mode instead of focusing on the matter they wanted to address. Managing misused diversion is not about ignoring trauma and pain, it is about finding ways forward that allow for problems to be resolved respectfully, fairly and equitably.

Diversion may also be used to shift a person's attention away to a seemingly more immediate or dramatic concern about someone else. This kind of deflection works well when it is used to target someone's interests, vulnerabilities, or sensitivities. It can be used blatantly or subtly. For example, you

4. Denial. It's not just a river in Africa.

might raise a concern about your partner's drinking levels, but they then mention they are worried about your teenage son. As a caring parent, you quickly become absorbed in wanting to help the child rather than dealing with your partner who diverted your focus away from them.

Diversion can be used as a sophisticated victim role or poor-me tactic that guarantees the person who is in denial of their own problems or bad behaviour does not have to change. At its worst, diversion may become gaslighting, a toxic and dangerous strategy employed by people who wish to manipulate others into doubting themselves and questioning their own sanity. Gaslighting involves lying, telling you that you did or did not do something and when your memory is different, someone who is gaslighting you can make you question the validity of your own memory. They can make problems someone else's responsibility and never take any blame. They can make you question your perception of events and lead you into feeling guilty, bad, at fault or responsible for things you are not actually responsible for. Whilst some gaslighting behaviour may have its roots in real trauma, or someone who uses diversion has a genuinely tough history, it might be valuable to acknowledge that **mental health is never an excuse for abuse** and if there are genuine reasons behind unhelpful or harmful behaviour these are the responsibility of the individual to address. Problems are better off being managed and addressed, not diverted onto someone else through avoiding personal responsibility, acting disrespectfully, or perpetrating abuse or violence.

Distraction

Distraction can also be a helpful coping mechanism when we

are facing a situation that we can do very little or nothing about at the time. It allows us to land in another space for a short while, to take some of the burden or stress and strain off our shoulders. It is usually only successful in the short-term because whatever we are facing is more than likely causing such distress that it cannot be covered up either completely or permanently. But, used sparingly and consciously, distraction can help us ride through situations until some kind of resolution can be found.

On those occasions where we are being faced with an overwhelming emotional experience and we have neither the space or support to deal with it, distraction and diversion can allow us to maintain a level of coping until either more resources can be found, or we have space to deal with our feelings. For example, it might not be helpful to have a meltdown at work when something has triggered you. Either distracting yourself with some kind of conscious movement or diverting into another work-related task that you can do something about can be a helpful short-term strategy to allow you to get through the day until you can get home, where you can then seek the help and support you need or allow yourself to feel your emotions in a safer space. Distraction is not a long-term solution. Distracting yourself constantly may lead you back into denial, and ignoring that there is a problem so that you avoid the emotions you are experiencing.

Another facet found in the tactic of distraction is achieved through unconscious dissociating. This is the act of involuntarily removing yourself from being in touch with your feelings or even your body to avoid dealing with something that feels too big or too much to handle. This occurs as a protective mechanism, often seen in response to childhood trauma. It can be unconsciously employed by the brain without you realising it as a way of shielding you from attack, harm or being

4. Denial. It's not just a river in Africa.

overwhelmed. After serious, repeated trauma, this can become an automated response to any threat (real or perceived), which can then be problematic for a number of reasons. The danger is that the feelings can continue to build and escalate, then overwhelm you, usually at an inappropriate time or in a more damaging way. If you dissociate in non-threatening environments, you could miss out on useful information being shared pertaining to your relationships, job, or children. It could make you inattentive of what you are doing, such as leaving something on the stove to burn, or tripping over an unseen hazard as you are not fully present. It may be that you consider seeking help to manage dissociation so it can be approached carefully and positively, and you may need professional assistance to do this.

Avoidance

Avoidance essentially underpins the other three unhelpful strategies. Denial is avoiding admitting that there is a problem. Diversion may allow us to avoid making changes or delaying dealing with an issue or by-passing responsibility onto someone else who then has to change instead of us. Distraction allows us to avoid feeling the problem while doing something else. Avoidance is blatantly not dealing with an issue. We can make ourselves very busy. We can avoid the person we may have an issue with. We can outrightly refuse to discuss or deal with the matter without any excuse or reason being given.

Avoidance changes nothing because nothing is being addressed. The problem will continue, and uncomfortable emotions associated with the issue fester and build. The more we avoid it, the bigger the mountain can seem to climb, to the point of absolute terror for some. We can then oscillate between the fight, flight, and freeze modes and avoidance becomes about survival, as dealing with the issue now seems overwhelmingly frightening and that fear then immobilises us completely. It is less risky to avoid the matter than to chance dealing with it. Avoidance is most definitely not a helpful coping mode and is best avoided (pun intended).

Managing Avoidance

Developing insight into how we might overuse and interact with these tools to avoid problems, avoid our feelings, avoid change, or avoid being challenged is part of our positive emotional coping strategy. Through honesty with ourselves and our observations, we can establish what tendencies we have to utilise these four techniques, and assess if we are overusing them and avoiding our avoidance, and then we can make adjustments accordingly. Once we can observe the overuse or misuse of these coping tools in ourselves, we may also become more adept at spotting them in others. This is particularly useful when you need to be attentive to those who might try to manipulate you or even gaslight you. If you can spot someone trying to make you feel like you are the one in the wrong or perpetrating the unwanted behaviour instead of them or make you responsible for something that they must address or even tries to make you question your own sense of reality, then you can either address the situation with the person and if they cannot safely engage in a dialogue with you, you may need to remove this person from your life and manage the situation from a place of awareness and clarity of what they are attempting to do to you.

There is a wide spectrum of manipulative behaviours that

4. Denial. It's not just a river in Africa.

we can observe frequently in society, ranging from small twists of the truth to avoid responsibility, to very damaging psychological and emotional abuse. Being able to identify when this is occurring is helpful in supporting and protecting our wellbeing and our safety. When we observe unhelpful behaviour and manipulations, we have an opportunity to be in control of how we respond. When we do not observe them and remain oblivious, we may end up very much not in control and therefore maybe more vulnerable to being manipulated and hurt. Take the time to understand how you use these 4 coping modes and take the time to see them in others. It may help serve to protect you and help to build better relationships through healthier dialogues that are based around managing problems, not avoiding them.

Exercise: Your Emotional Coping Pie

Have a think about the 4 potentially unhelpful coping mechanisms and think about where you might use them.

1. Ask yourself, do you use them briefly or over long periods? For example, a drink at the end of the week is not going to risk your liver too much. But drinking a 6-pack or a bottle of wine every day to avoid feeling bad is.

2. Write down situations where you try to avoid either feeling a certain way or dealing with a problem. Is this helpful or harmful? For instance, not talking to your partner because you feel uncomfortable won't help your relationship over the long-term. Taking time to get some guidance from a friend or therapist and then approaching your partner could help support you into more conducive forms of communication.

3. Are there things you feel guilty about that stop you from looking at yourself? Believing everyone else must be looked after first can lead to you to being burned out and drained. Blaming other people or situations for your emotional state is not helpful and might prevent

4. Denial. It's not just a river in Africa.

you from putting your emotional wellbeing back under your control.

4. Are you afraid of change, or of yourself? Do you get angry when you are frightened or feel guilty? What are your fears about dealing with your emotions? Do you fear you could become overwhelmed if you start feeling your feelings and you could lose control? Do you worry how others may perceive you if you admit fault, or fear they could take advantage of you?

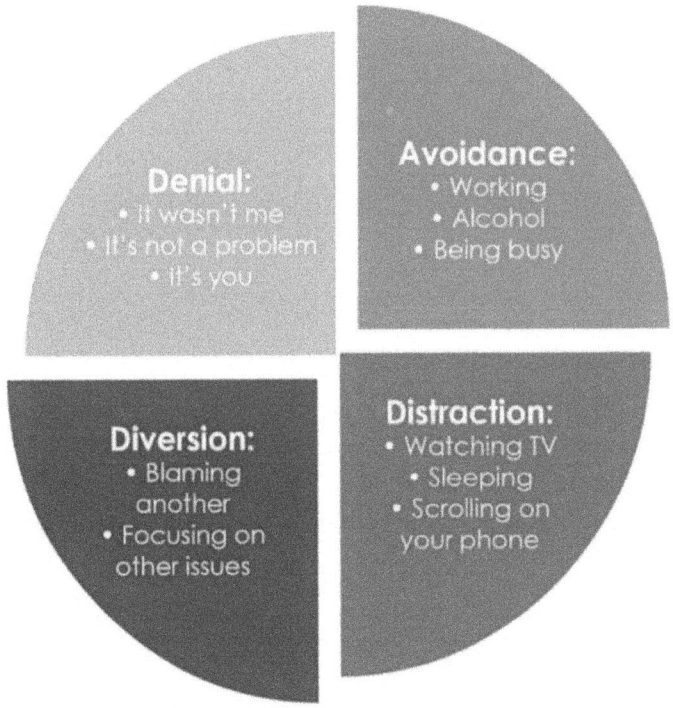

Maybe use the diagram here as a guide to help you work out what kinds of strategies you use to cope and how often you use them. What does you pie look like? Are you using too much distraction that it's become unhelpful? Is denial helping you fight against something or stopping you from dealing with things? Is diversion delaying the issue too much? Is avoidance making the initial problem grow bigger in your mind?

If you find this exercise brings up difficult emotions, please pause and consider seeking support from a therapist or mental health professional.

4. Denial. It's not just a river in Africa.

Pause—Reflect—Landscape

1. **Pause** - Take a moment to sit with what you have just learned and consider it.

- There are 4 types of coping mechanisms that if we overuse them, they can become damaging and harmful, possibly affecting our own wellbeing, our relationships and the safety of ourselves and others.
- Denial can be a source of strength and resilience used to overcome obstacles. But it can become an avoidance that there is a problem that would be better off being addressed.
- Diversion can be used to move our attention elsewhere to build confidence, find comfort or experience lighter emotions to either create some respite from the uncomfortable emotions or delay dealing with an issue until a more appropriate time. Or it can be used to shift the focus off the issue and even onto someone else, passing responsibility off and meaning nothing is potentially getting resolved.
- Distraction is about changing our feelings or our focus to not have to face a situation or feel pain. But this could

go on too long and may cause the original emotional injury to fester and worsen.

- Avoidance is the refusal to engage or deal with the feelings or problems at hand.

- Being aware of which ones we use and choosing how little or often we employ these tools may help protect us from overuse and minimise future risk or risk of harm to ourselves and others.

2. **Reflect** - Answer the following questions:

   - How have you felt whilst reading about these 4 coping tools, did recognise either your own or others behaviour in any of them?

   - Do you see any risks to overusing these tools in your life or risks from other people around you who might overuse them?

   - Would you be willing to look at changing how you use any of these tools? How could you approach or manage other people who overuse these tools?

3. **Landscape** - Step back from the details and see how this new information fits in with the bigger picture of your life. Consider your history, what is going on for you now, who and what is in your life, and the future you want for yourself.

   → When you look back over your life can you see relationships or situations that were not helped by you or others overusing any of these 4 coping tools? Did these tools block you from changing or prevent you from maintaining good new habits?

4. Denial. It's not just a river in Africa.

→ Do you have ideas on how you could balance accessing the positive utility of these tools and maintaining an awareness of their effects to reduce risks of overuse? What alternative coping methods could use instead of them?

→ Do you have any unhelpful beliefs that make you doubt your own capacity, or do you have low self-worth that feeds into you over accessing these tools to avoid your feelings or responsibilities?

5. It Wasn't Me! Managing the Intrusion of Guilt and Influence of Fear

In this section you will be learning about:

- → Why do we want to avoid feeling guilty?
- → How can intention and self-kindness help us in managing guilt?
- → How does fear underlie many of our uncomfortable feelings?
- → How we can build a strategy to manage guilt and fear more healthily.

You will need:

- ✓ A positive attitude towards changing.
- ✓ To show kindness towards yourself for things that do not serve you.
- ✓ Openness to using guilt as an opportunity for change and growth.
- ✓ To make notes on any insights that arise.
- ✓ To be open to discussing your reactions, feelings, and ideas, either with yourself or others.

5. It Wasn't Me! Managing the Intrusion of Guilt and Influence of Fear

"Avoiding danger is no safer in the long run than outright exposure. The fearful are caught as often as the bold."

Helen Keller

One emotion most people will happily avoid is guilt. Of the myriad emotions that we encounter, guilt can be one of the most difficult. With most of the other emotions, we might be more likely to allow ourselves to feel them and process them, and we may find it easier to let them go and move forward. Guilt, on the other hand, can cause us to linger in the moment that has passed and trap us in the unsolvable quandary of "if only", or "I should have known better", potentially causing us to feel excessive anger, disappointment, negative self-judgment and fear—all of which can, potentially, leave us vulnerable to other problems. As the past does not exist anymore, we cannot change what has happened, ruminating over the mistake we cannot alter does not serve us. An example of this might be the distracted individual who reverses into another car and feels terrible for causing an accident, but keeps ruminating, thinking "if only I was paying more attention". The more they think about what they could have done, the less present they are, distracted by the unchangeable past mistake, and ironically putting themselves at risk of another accident because they are not paying attention to their present.

Guilt can feel deeply uncomfortable, it can lead us into damaging negative self-narratives, where we may become hypercritical of ourselves, and we risk lowering our self-esteem, maybe we end up believing we are not worthy of good things or even deserve punishment. Guilt can reduce our self-confidence, create doubt in our capacity, and lead us into a vulnerable state where we are likely to make more mistakes. Guilt can become a major roadblock to change as it remains solely positioned in an unalterable past. The guilt spiral generally goes nowhere good.

We can feel guilty in a multitude of ways, it isn't just when we've made a mistake or done something wrong. It could be when we don't spend enough time with those we love. We may feel guilty asking something of someone who we know is already struggling with their own burdens. We could experience guilt when we didn't do what we said we would do. We may feel guilty for hiding something from someone. Guilty for being late. Guilty for taking care of ourselves, or prioritising ourselves. Guilt and perfectionism can also align unhealthily for us when we set ourselves an unreasonable target that we fall short of. More worrisome is when other people can use our propensity for guilt to manipulate us. They might tap into our willingness to avoid guilt and use this to leverage us into meeting their needs and following their agenda. This could drain our personal finite resources, be it our energy, time, skills, or money, even putting us into possibly abusive situations and trapping us in unhealthy relationships.

Guilt can become singularly focused on the moment that

5. It Wasn't Me! Managing the Intrusion of Guilt and Influence of Fear

we feel guilty about and does not always allow for reconstruction, reframing, or growth. This can make it one of the least useful uncomfortable emotions when it falls down this particular spiral. Developing a strategy on how to manage guilt could be extremely confronting. It requires acknowledging things about us that we might not like, and we may have to let go of things that are helping us avoid making the changes we fear. Because guilt can enter our lives in so many ways, from the small to the large, to the potentially dangerous if used by someone who is manipulating us, it makes it even more relevant that we continue to seek ways in which we might resolve and manage guilt more quickly and efficiently. A good starting place for managing guilt is to invest time into thinking about the relationship you have with guilt, how it works within your structure of coping, and how it plays out in your life:

- Are you someone who feels guilty?
- Do you avoid it?
- Can you get bogged down in thinking you could have, would have, should have type thinking?
- How do you resolve guilt?
- Do you deal with your guilt or bury it?

Managing guilt is another step toward creating your psychodiversity and may enable you to adapt and sustain through the inevitably guilty moments that crop up in our lives.

Hindsight bias and guilt can have a close relationship that might make us feel uncomfortable. Hindsight bias can provide us with the illusion that our decisions are good or bad based on the outcome, regardless of the process we undertook to make the decision or the information available to us at the time the decision was made. We may try to convince ourselves that we should have known better or could have done more, but only after the outcome has happened. Basing judgment of a decision only on the outcome can be a flawed process and likely to make us believe something impossible, that we can always predict the exact outcome. It is not an absolute truth that we will always be able to see what will come of our decisions every time. You could, for example, with all the best intentions in the world and careful planning, prepare a beautiful meal for someone special to you, but amid your excitement of doing something nice and an unexpected trip to the vet for your dog, you forgot that this was a night they had planned with their friends, and they are upset you didn't remember. Or you prepared a report at work, and despite being tired and overworked, you thought you did a great job. But after you submit it, you find that a piece of information is now wrong because, unbeknownst to you, the situation changed and no one told you, and that has now caused a problem for someone else to deal with. Outcomes are at times not under our complete control and can be affected by numerous factors beyond our choices and influence. This means that if we expect an outcome to be assured solely based on our own information and actions, hindsight bias may hoodwink us into believing that an unexpected result is entirely our fault. This, in turn, can trigger unhelpful and uncomfortable emotional experiences.

If we are using our emotions as informants, what does guilt tell us? Breaking this emotion down and understanding what we can learn from events can gain us practical and serviceable knowledge that may then guide us into making different choices in the future. When learning is extrapolated, we have a greater opportunity for making more sustainable decisions that

5. It Wasn't Me! Managing the Intrusion of Guilt and Influence of Fear

could create better emotional outcomes for us later down the track. When we have caused hurt to another person or created a difficult situation for others, then it is understandable and very human to feel guilty. It can be a positive sign because it may mean you care about others and wish to do no harm. That is a strength. So, rather than remaining in guilt, perhaps by acknowledging that you feel bad and understanding that it at least shows you care, you can move from the stagnant space of "if only" to being in the dynamic and more productive energy of "I can be better next time, or I can be more careful because I care."

Compromising your capacity to function and lowering your self-esteem through ruminating on guilty feelings is not going to serve you or anyone else. Make guilt serviceable, and turn it into something useful to you and others. Feeling bad for making mistakes is OK; it means you care, have empathy, and want to do better. None of these are undesirable traits. They are all useful, positive qualities. You cannot undo the past, but you certainly can change in the present and strive for better in the future.

Fear - Our Friend or Foe?

One of the emotions underpinning our avoidant coping mechanisms, blocking change and feeding guilt is our old frenemy, fear. When we are afraid change is unlikely to be supported, welcomed or maintained as fear can paralyse us, trapping us into a frozen state where any action feels too risky or too much. But fear, believe it or not, can sometimes be our friend. By seeing it thus, it may allow us to make friends with some of our fears and nurture them with compassion. It means you accept rather than deny your fears, and therefore you can do something about them, even if it is just supporting yourself actively with care and kindness whilst you are feeling afraid. If fear becomes your foe, you end up fearing your fear, which may not be a good space to be in.

Whether we are avoiding our feelings or stuck in guilt, it can be because we are feeling frightened. We may be frightened by our emotions, frightened by what we have done, frightened by how we might appear to others, frightened of what might happen if we change or allow ourselves to feel pain and discomfort, what if the pain never stops? We could fear consequences and even carry trauma from being punished unfairly in the past. We may be frightened we might not be good enough to change or cope. There are lots of potential ways for fear to creep in. To find a way through guilt and stop avoiding, it may help us to become more intimate with our fears and then use our strengths to face them. But confronting our fears is something we can all find very hard to do.

Many of us use fear as the foundation to build protective walls around ourselves and others as way to minimise risk and avert pain. Someone who has been hurt before in a past relationship might keep others then at a distance, fearing being hurt again. Or we might avoid taking up opportunities or trying new things due to previous bad experiences that have harmed or frightened us. But this kind of protective avoidance is not necessarily a strategy that is sustainable, and we may still end up hurt or feeling bad anyway for missing out. Boxing ourselves in does not allow us to see the breadth of what we have and can offer, both to ourselves and others. Mistakes and bad experiences happen; it may help not to make a second mistake by becoming stuck in a past you cannot alter.

Moving to intent can be a positive way out of avoidance and

5. It Wasn't Me! Managing the Intrusion of Guilt and Influence of Fear

guilt, and ultimately in dealing with fear. Did you intend to shut yourself off from the good things? Did you intend to shut out other people for so long? Did you intend to hurt someone? Did you plan it meticulously? Were you sitting up in bed the night before making a list of how you could hurt that person? Hopefully, the answer to these questions is no. Generally, we do not set out to deliberately curtail or hurt either ourselves or another person. But we can unconsciously be trying to protect ourselves or even be a bit mindless at times and make judgment calls that do not work out. We can react badly out of pain and trauma, or we can make genuine mistakes due to fatigue, confusion, or misreading a situation. But these things can be managed and addressed with gentle care, compassion, and sometimes professional help. We can learn to be more mindful and considerate of ourselves and others. We can ask for clarification of a situation before responding. We can ensure we look after ourselves to manage fatigue or pain. We can slow down our reactions and consider for a moment, before using a possibly hurtful retort in retaliation. We can seek help to heal trauma that may be creating fears and causing us to use protections that stop us from living our lives.

Intention may ease guilt and soften fear and help you identify workable solutions to a situation. Do not get confused with actions that go wrong and the definition of your character. It is all too easy to say, I am a bad person or that's typical of me, I always get it wrong. These types of negative statements may make you seem like a victim of your past or that you are naturally a bad person, making you possibly feel this is something you can do nothing about, so it's ok to give up on yourself. But that's probably not true. Once we come to terms with our intentions and have been able to forgive our actions, we may find that we can apologise where needed to start the process of making amends with others, and then by changing our actions and behaviours we may find we can rebuild trust. Saying the words sometimes can be the easier part of the healing process. Changing is likely to require you to carefully and gently face your fears about yourself. Learning to compassionately let go of the "I am such a terrible person" idea or the "it's not my fault" attitude and recognising that your actions may be part of the problem, means you can place your behaviour back under your control—and thus, it can be gradually changed.

Fear can be our friend when we view it as being a supportive part of our functioning, it may aid us to make informed decisions and help us take educated or calculated risks to keep ourselves safe at times. Fear may serve us and support our intuition. But fear can also undo us. Many of our uncomfortable emotions link back to fear. Understanding the nature of fear and how it manifests within us may help us towards developing a deeper understanding about those uncomfortable emotions so we might transmute them. For example, we can be angry because we are afraid. We are afraid of something happening or of something not happening. Envy and jealousy can be about the fear of not having something or of not getting to experience something. Boredom can be about being afraid of being alone with ourselves and our thoughts, our self-phobia. We can be feeling fear without even recognising it or understanding what we are afraid of. Our fear may sit in the realm of the ego, and the ego works with labels and absolutes, and is not always a friend of nuance. Using our awareness, we can attempt to strip back the layers of emotion, to seek out the nuances, the subtleties and details of what is going on inside that fear, all from a backdrop of understanding how our fear

5. It Wasn't Me! Managing the Intrusion of Guilt and Influence of Fear

presents an inviting, though daunting, opportunity to get to know ourselves better.

Let's revisit that acronym of fear, False Evidence Appearing Real. Fear can be about a future that has not happened, but that could happen. It can be about what-ifs. Understanding time in relation to your feeling of fear may support you in dealing with it differently. By facing your fears, you can work out exactly what they are about, and ascertain if it is a real-live, happening now threat or something that could happen one day kind of threat, and this gives you a roadmap to potentially managing them. For example, when you are afraid of something happening in the future, there may be many steps that could be taken or avoided that might alter the outcome. Thinking about your potential options could reduce or minimise, the fear. Reassuring yourself that you can cope well, and you can find a way through it and that you have your own back may support you in feeling more capable. Having confidence and finding strength in your up-to-now survival stats (that is you've made it through this far) could aid in reducing feelings of fear and encouraging an attitude of **"I've got this"**. Remember that making absolutes your future is not always reality, sometimes fear is just an illusion of what could be.

Getting caught in what has happened in the past often seems like a guarantee it is going to happen again. Life does not always work like this. Whilst repetition is always possible, it is never a sure thing, that is a relative truth, not an absolute truth. Focusing on what has happened could stop you from paying attention to the present, where you may have an opportunity to change or even alter the trajectory of the scenario you are worried about. Contextualising your fear in terms of the timeframe can be a helpful way of managing it. Using thinking that reminds you that you have coped with problems before and come through it, you can do again, creates a much more supportive mindset than succumbing to overwhelming fears of not being able to cope that could stall you into freeze mode and keep you trapped in that uncomfortable space for far too long.

Consider becoming more intimate with your fears and comforting yourself though them. They are not to be negatively judged. Embrace and ease yourself through them to a place of **"I can seek ways to cope, no matter what."** Set yourself up in a mindset of positive support by acknowledging that when you are afraid, that perhaps it is OK to be afraid, and that you can continue to look after yourself in managing this fear and seeking solutions or opportunities to either alleviate or eradicate the source of it. Go gently and kindly, this can be intense work.

Fear and Guilt Management Protocol:

Getting help with the potentially disabling and detrimental effects created by both guilt and fear seems only logical and by developing a protocol to manage both we may be able to care for and protect ourselves appropriately. They are inevitable human experiences, we will all be exposed to at different times, by knowing how we interact with these emotions and what problems they could cause for us if not being actively overseen is what this protocol can support you in managing.

The protocol includes the when, the why, the what and the how. The when is about identifying situations you're likely to experience guilt or fear. The why is about recognising the beliefs and values that could make you vulnerable to guilt and drive your fears. The what component reveals and isolates the basis of your fears and what might be sitting beneath that guilt, or your avoidance in any given situation. The how is about the solutions and potential changes you could make to accept and support yourself, make amends where relevant, and create solutions to support you now and your future self from repeating mistakes and keeping fears manageable so they do not block change, limit your life or potential, and may even limit the time you spend feeling emotionally uncomfortable.

1. **When:**
    - When do you feel guilty? What behaviours do you have that make you feel bad?
    - When do you get scared? In what situations might fear become a factor for you?
    - Does hindsight bias cloud your judgment at times, making you think you should have known more, done more and been more? Is this a relative truth or absolute truth?

2. **Why:**
    - Does your experience of guilt correlate with your values? For example, were you taught to put others first? Or do you believe you must always do everything perfectly?
    - Do your beliefs create opportunities for fear to influence you? For instance, if you have low self-worth, does this then make you more nervous or afraid when you have to take on new or demanding tasks?
    - Look back at the beliefs and values you have isolated so far in this journey, see if anything could leave you susceptible to feeling guilty or opens the doorway to creating fear.

3. **What:**
    - What are you afraid of when you avoid feeling guilty or any of your emotions?
    - Recriminations? Consequences? Payback? Being unpopular or disliked? Being told off or feeling embarrassed?
    - Do past experiences drive your fears or make you feel guilty?
    - What is your fear about, something that has happened, something that is happening now, or something that could happen?
4. **How:**
    - How can your strengths help you with guilt or difficult emotional moments?
    - How did you set up your initial intentions, was it to get things wrong or cause harm? Could you soften your attitude towards yourself by looking at intentions as well as the outcome?
    - How can you change and support your current and future self to manage the negative spirals of shame and blame that could occur?
    - How can you implement solutions to help you avoid repeating incidents that cause you to feel guilty? Would it help to share these planned improvements to your behaviour with others?
    - How can you tell if someone is using guilt or fear to manipulate you?
    - How can you support yourself through guilt and fear to be more compassionate, kind and believe in your ability to grow from any experience?

Exercise: Fear and Guilt Management Protocol

You are going to experience the emotions of fear and guilt at some point in your life, so it seems to make sense to invest some time and energy into having a process for managing them.

Here are some preparatory questions that may help guide you into creating your own personal protocol around managing fear and guilt. Take your time answering these questions, some of them may be activating for you.

Maybe consider taking them to a professional therapist, counsellor, psychologist, or a trusted friend and work through them in a safe and supported environment. This is a deep reflective exercise that may not be appropriate to undertake without support, please consider use of this carefully in accordance with your own history and circumstances.

Apologising:

1. Can I admit when I have made a mistake, or do I feel ashamed, foolish, or angry at myself?

2. Would my perception of how I view mistakes benefit from being changed to be a more positive experience?

3. How easy do I find apologising? Do I apologise too much? Is it hard for me?
4. Do I fear being negatively judged and excluded? Do I fear I look weak or become a target? Do I fear being manipulated or gaslit? Do I excessively worry about harming or hurting others?
5. If I fear being honest and apologetic with others, are there ways I can protect myself, or are there people I could let go of or distance myself from if I cannot safely take accountability with them?

Facing the fear:

1. Do I feel afraid when I feel guilty? Am I afraid of owning my error in case I get in more trouble? Do I fear how others might judge me? Do I judge myself harshly?
2. If I openly own my mistakes, can I still trust myself and know I had good intentions, and not let someone bully me or take advantage of me?
3. How do I cope with feeling scared? What actions do I take, or behaviours do I have when I feel afraid?
4. Can I dig in behind my fear to see if there is an unhelpful belief that is driving this fear? Can I see if my fear or this belief is relative truth or an absolute truth? Can I reframe this belief to be more supportive for managing fear?

Self-compassion:

1. Would developing more self-compassion when I get something wrong, help me to feel safer and less afraid to own my mistakes and then be able to make amends and changes?

5. It Wasn't Me! Managing the Intrusion of Guilt and Influence of Fear

2. Do I feel like my self-worth is lessened because I acknowledge something I did wrong? Would it help to show kindness to myself and recall that I am more than one moment or one choice?

3. What is the best way for me to feel comfortable when I am dealing with uncomfortable emotions? Could I reassure myself in my mind that I am human, that mistakes happen, and that I can always learn from them and do better next time? Would it help to acknowledge my fear and validate that it's ok to be afraid, and then find a way to support myself into feeling safer and calmer?

Using your reflections from the questions above, you are invited to explore how you might build a personal strategy for responding to feelings of fear and guilt. This reflective activity may support you in identifying when and why these emotions arise, what is sitting behind them and how you can action approaches that might be helpful for your unique personality, values, and life experience. You might also consider speaking with others about how they navigate fear or guilt. Hearing a range of perspectives may help you discover additional ideas that feel relevant or supportive to your process.

Once you've created a strategy or set of supportive steps, you may find it helpful to revisit and reflect on them regularly. Repetition and gentle reinforcement can play a role in strengthening your ability to access helpful coping strategies over time. If you notice that particular tools are working well for you, practising them consistently may gradually increase your confidence and ability to respond effectively in emotionally challenging situations. While meaningful change often takes time and sustained effort, the process of learning new emotional skills can contribute to greater resilience and a stronger sense of self-support.

This could be an intense and activating exercise, and you may consider reading it through first before commencing and deciding if this might better approached alongside a professional therapist.

1. **When can I feel guilty or afraid?**

    - Write down some of the times you have felt guilty or been afraid, maybe include situations that you know could make you feel guilty and fearful.
    - Perhaps include times when other people have made you feel guilty for your actions or behaviour.
    - Look out for the appearance of hindsight bias that might try to trick you into thinking you could have controlled all the factors that influenced the outcome of a situation.

    This information may help prepare you to become more aware of the times you are likely to experience guilt and fear so you can be ready you help yourself through the emotions.

    Example: I can feel guilty or afraid when I think I have hurt or upset people, or if I let anyone down. I am afraid they might leave me or exclude me. People have taken advantage of this to get me to do more for them.

2. **Why do I feel guilty or afraid?**

    - Look back over your beliefs and values from your earlier work. Find out which ones may lead you into feeling guilty and which ones might lead you into being fearful.

- Perhaps when you notice you are feeling guilty, you could ask yourself which belief or value is influencing this feeling?
- If you are afraid, ask yourself is this a fear of something that has happened, is happening or might happen?

By adjusting or softening any unhelpful beliefs or values you could help ease the guilt, and support the fear so it does not overwhelm you, and you may stop yourself from spiralling into shame or blame dynamics to find some solutions to move forward with.

Example: I value being caring and putting others first. I always must do my best and get things right. I hate being alone or left out.

If we deceive ourselves by either believing a negative or positive attribute that isn't true, we could limit our capacity to change or overcome challenges. I can learn to enjoy my own company and make my own fun or find new friends, rather than doing things for others just to keep their friendship.

3. **What am I afraid of in this situation?**
    - Are there things that you fear might happen when something goes wrong?
    - Are there things you fear that might not happen?
    - Do certain situations remind you of an experience where you were manipulated or punished unfairly? Can you make yourself more present so you can fairly assess if it is happening again without being overwhelmed or biased by your fear?

Compassionately looking at your guilt, and gently supporting yourself to look at your fears, may help you to deconstruct what is really going on for you. This knowledge could then support you in addressing the situation and comforting yourself towards positive resolution and change.

Example: I am afraid other people will think less of me if I do a bad job. I am afraid I won't be included if people think I am not good enough. I am afraid to lose people I love if I hurt them. I lost a previous relationship and this hurt me deeply. This can be a vulnerability for me because someone who wants to control me could use my fear of them leaving to get me to do what they want. I can care kindly for myself, seek help when needed and trust that if I lose some relationships, I can learn from them and create others.

4. **How can I help myself move out of guilt into reconciliation, change or letting go?**

    - What can you kindly acknowledge about the guilt you experience?

    - What was your intention in the situation? What are the positives in this situation?

    - How it would feel to apologise to yourself or others, and what is the safest way to do this?

    - What actions can you take to show you have learned from the situation?

    - Could you consider how to protect yourself from someone who's using guilt or fear to manipulate you?

Put together the information of the when, the why, and the what to see how you could support yourself in managing fear and guilt more safely, and compassionately.

5. It Wasn't Me! Managing the Intrusion of Guilt and Influence of Fear

Example: Worrying about hurting others indicates I am a good person; my intention is to help not harm. This shows me a strength not a weakness. I can apologise to others for my part but it is equally important I recognise their role in the situation to help prevent me from being taken advantage of. I can be kinder to myself when things don't go as planned or I make a mistake and find ways to be more comfortable balancing putting myself first at times, above others. I value myself, what I have to give and wish to find others who treat me as I treat them.

If you find this exercise brings up difficult emotions, please pause and consider seeking support from a therapist or mental health professional.

Pause — Reflect — Landscape

1. **Pause** - Take a moment to sit with what you have just learned and consider it.

- Guilt may trap us in a past we can't change and may then put us at risk of repeating past mistakes in the present. Guilt can be uncomfortable, and we may naturally want to avoid it, but this means we might not take responsibility appropriately, and this could negatively affect us and our relationships.

- Hindsight bias can trick us into thinking we could have done more or should have known better, even when all the factors that can influence an outcome are not under our control.

- Fear can underlie guilt and stop us taking responsibility, apologising or changing.

- Asking what our guilt is telling us may help us to manage it and reframe the emotion into an opportunity for managing the situation and cultivating personal growth. Finding strength in our guilt can help us to feel brave to face our fears or make amends and do better in the future.

5. It Wasn't Me! Managing the Intrusion of Guilt and Influence of Fear

- Looking at our intention may help us to assuage our guilt and may allow us to move forward to reconciliation and future improvements.

- Fear is both useful and detrimental to us, and facing our fears could support us in finding out whether our fear is helpful or harmful in a situation. Using fear to protect ourselves may not be helpful, effective or sustainable.

- Establishing if our fear is about something happening now, something from the past repeating, or something in the future can help us to manage it. By using the relative and absolute truth equation we might lessen the load of fear and see ways to help ourselves and opportunities to challenge our fears.

- Having a fear and guilt management protocol may help us cope in guilty moments and could assist us in supporting ourselves when we feel frightened.

2. **Reflect** - Answer the following questions:

    - Are you someone who can ruminate on mistakes? Over apologise? Or are you the opposite and avoid guilt by denying you were any part of the problem or blaming others? Is apologising hard for you, and if yes why?

    - Do you carry a lot of guilt, or have you been manipulated into taking too much responsibility and this still causes you problems? Is this something you could seek help with from a professional?

    - Is fear a dominant emotion in your life? Does it stop you achieving your goals or realising your dreams? Do you manage your fear, or does it manage you?

3. **Landscape** - Step back from the details and see how this new information fits in with the bigger picture of your life. Consider your history, what is going on for you now, who and what is in your life, and the future you want for yourself.

- ✓ Can you see times in your life when fear or guilt have affected your openness to change? Stopped you from being able to enter or maintain a change process? Or held you back from completing your goals?
- ✓ Can you identify any blocks to you implementing a fear and guilt management protocol that could help you now and on the longer term? This might include past experiences, concerns about how others see you, or fears you might drop your own standards and start failing as a result. What can you do to remove any blocks you find?
- ✓ Is it possible that whilst you think you take responsibility in situations, you do this by putting more blame onto others, making yourself look less guilty to feel better about yourself?
- ✓ Has trauma influenced how guilt or fear shows up in your life? Or exacerbated or worsened these two challenging emotional experiences? Is this an area where you might need to access some professional specialised trauma therapy?

6. Positive Emotional Coping

In this section you will be learning about:

- → How can mindfulness support and underpin positive emotional coping?
- → Why it may be helpful to manage our judgment of our emotional experiences?
- → What are the steps necessary for positive emotional coping?

You will need:

- ✓ A space to reflect and carry out a written exercise.
- ✓ To acknowledge this may be uncomfortable and to show yourself compassion.
- ✓ To remember feelings are temporary.
- ✓ Pen and paper to make notes on any insights that arise.
- ✓ To be open to discussing your reactions, feelings, and ideas, either with yourself or others.

6. Positive Emotional Coping

"I choose not to think of my life as surviving but coping."
                                               Lorna Luft

From our explorations into our emotions, we have learned that they can act as agents of information. We can avoid our feelings by overusing certain coping mechanisms, and we have seen how guilt and fear might block our openness to change. By now, it is likely becoming apparent how our emotional wellbeing, our ability to manage our feelings and our awareness of what they signal, can have a direct and profound impact on our ability to undertake and sustain change. Without insight and a set of reliable tools to manage our emotional coping capacity, we can veer into avoidance, which does not permit for any kind of change, we can be hindered by guilt and halted by fear. Boredom and impatience might create unhelpful feelings of frustration that could derail our attempts at change and lead us back into previous behaviours or prior habits, without us even realising it has happened. Therefore, we can conclude that to support change and promote our growth, our psychodiversity would benefit from having a clear set of positive emotional coping skills and ways of managing our feelings that is both comfortable and tolerable.

A useful skill that can support you in your emotional management is being mindful. Mindfulness is about being present in all ways in the moment, paying attention to everything going on around you and inside of you. It can expand your capacity to calmly hear yourself and calmly make choices that suit the circumstances and may have the best possible impact in the future. Being mindful is the ability to listen in on yourself, so you can hear what your mind is cooking up. This skill may help you to hear your thoughts before you move into action, which allows you to assess if your planned behaviour may create scenarios that could trigger uncomfortable emotions or unwanted consequences. The better you get at listening to what your brain is doing when you are not fully conscious of it, the greater the opportunity you have to support yourself well. This may help you stop yourself setting up a situation that is going to do more harm than potential good. It's particularly useful for managing addictions and changing harmful habits. Just be aware that when you are dealing with trauma, mindfulness can be challenging to engage with and might not always be the right tool for the moment. We discuss this further in Book 3.

A component of the addiction pattern can be about the permissions and justifications that pave the way for the addictive habit and almost create support for it. Explanations are provided by the mind as to why the substance or behaviour is needed. These are taken as absolute truths by the unassuming subconscious and not questioned; thus, people can remain stuck, potentially repeating the unhelpful behaviour. Once we become mindfully aware of the permissions that we might be giving ourselves, we have a hope of challenging them and resisting them. We have the chance to see through the stories that we are telling ourselves that allow us to use the harmful substance or perform the unhelpful behaviour again. We can see beyond the moment that we are in and into the future by using another part of our mind. Then, by stretching forward to

6. Positive Emotional Coping

the future and looking back at the past, we may see what we are doing has caused us harm before and how it might do us harm in the future. Therefore, the suggestion could be that a better decision in the present might be wise. This isn't to flippantly say that being mindful fixes addictions, it is much more complicated than that, but it is a skill that can be supportive when overcoming them.

Dealing with our uncomfortable emotions, as we know, is not always pretty. It can be painful and hard to bear at times. There can be understandable reasons we use avoidant patterns of coping as previously discussed in chapter 4: feeling our feelings can hurt. But, fortunately, they are part of our human existence. Without them, we might not recognise when we are happy or content. We might not grow and challenge and change ourselves to become greater than what we were. They are necessary, and potentially useful. For example, when we experience the loss of love, after allowing ourselves to feel those uncomfortable emotions of sadness, disappointment and hurt we may then see afterwards that the depth of our pain mirrors how deep and valuable that love was, and that perhaps we were fortunate to experience such a love, as some might not. When we find love again, we may then potentially have an even greater experience from this space of recognition and appreciation that the uncomfortable emotions afforded us.

No one is saying that dealing with your emotions is going to be a straightforward or simple task. It is very much not easy, especially when you carry trauma. But when you find ways to develop skills that support you to be comfortable being uncomfortable, when you learn how to accept that these feelings are valid and any person in that situation would more than likely feel the exact same way, and that their intensity can be temporary, then you may well find you are more open to acknowledging your feelings and be ready to deal with them, without unfairly judging yourself or blocking the attempt. When you allow yourself to feel the emotions, and contextualise why they are there, then you might be able to establish whether there is something you can do about them or a perspective that you can reframe to alter how you are feeling or simply support yourself in that moment. It may be, at times, the situation is something that you just have to accept and cope with as best you can until it runs its course. But the intensity of all feelings is temporary. If the comfortable ones don't last, it stands to reason the uncomfortable ones won't either. Acknowledging that some emotional experiences, particularly ones pertaining to grief for example, may work somewhat differently. The feeling of grief may never be fully resolved or pass, but how we manage it, the intensity of it and refining the way we move out of it can change with time and from gaining experience in handling ourselves with care through those moments of loss.

Whilst we may try to hide or suppress our feelings, they can have a way of popping out of us whether we like it or not. Being prepared to deal with them through a safe and supportive structure that we purposely create within ourselves may assist us in managing our emotional experience well. If you are dealing with trauma, it may make the process feel more difficult. In these moments, being compassionate and kind towards yourself when managing your feelings could be supportive, and you may also find professional assistance helpful. Trauma can add another layer to coping, as it is such a personal and individual experience that varies from person to person. The impact of unregulated traumatic emotions may feel heavy across mental, emotional, physical, or spiritual aspects of life. If you are living with trauma, you might consider seeking professional support

6. Positive Emotional Coping

to explore approaches for emotional management. Having someone accompany you and support you on this journey may make all the difference.

We are going to discuss a three-part strategy you might consider using for your own positive emotional management, which consists of the stages **pause, process** and **progress**. The pause allows you recognise what you are feeling, it may be more than one emotion. The process is about feeling your feelings, letting the experience sit within and holding that space until it eases, not hiding it, not trying to distract from it but being with it, whether it shows up as an energy, movement, behaviour or feeling the actual feeling in the body. The progress is about how you move forward; what you might be able to learn, who might be good to communicate with and what you might use to help support yourself in the future.

Here are some ideas to help you start to evolve your own positive emotional framework, it does not need to look exactly like this, you may adapt these concepts to work in a healthy balance to align with your values and suit your style. Look over these and see if there are ones that feel more naturally comfortable than others. Are there ones you feel are too hard or too impossible to try? Can you look at why you feel that way, and ask yourself if this is connected to your beliefs about your capacity, and if it is, could you change this view of yourself? Talk them over with others and ask what they do. Invest time into thinking about them and using them in certain situations.

Some Preparatory Steps to Positive Emotional Coping

1. **List the feelings:**

   - Positive emotional coping is supported through the identification of all the feelings you experience pertaining to a situation. List them out and be ok if this takes a bit of time and support yourself with compassion if it is feeling quite hard to do.

   - Consider learning about the subtleties of emotions, the nuances, and find words to describe them. To do this more easily, you may benefit from educating yourself about the various types of emotion and what they might look and feel like for you.

2. **Look for the blocks:**

   - Identify and manage any blocks that you might have to coping with these feelings, such as fear or guilt.

   - Are there any unhelpful judgments you are holding, and are they absolute truths or relative truths?

   - Are you too busy to sit with your feelings right now? Or not in a safe place? Can you find a safe space to be with your feelings?

   - Do you need a professional to help you commence this journey into your feelings?

3. **Check your mindset:**

   - Assess whether you are in a problem-focused or solution-focused mindset. Are you describing the problem

6. Positive Emotional Coping

you are facing, or are you working out how you might deal with it and supporting yourself through it?

4. **Check which time zone your mind is in:**

    - Bring your awareness into the present and then consciously use your mind to look at the past, the present, and possible future. Have you been reminded of any past hurts? Are you worried about possible future hurts?

    - By shifting time zones, you can find information and possible solutions relevant to the current situation that may minimise uncomfortable emotions.

5. **Work with self-compassion, encouragement and support:**

    - Check-in: have you lapsed into a negative judgment against yourself, been harsh and critical? This may trigger other unhelpful past experiences where you have felt down about yourself and not good enough.

    - Move into a space where you do an assessment of the current situation that you are in through a compassionate and encouraging lens. Retain a perspective of self-compassion, being able to nurture yourself and treat yourself as you would a child or someone you cared deeply for who came to you and needed help.

    - When you approach yourself with this kind of gentle, compassionate, grounded surety, you can support yourself through the circumstance, with uncomfortable emotions potentially reducing or passing with more ease and care.

Once you have looked through this list of suggestions, identified any blocks and which approaches may work for you or adapted your own versions, you could trial the **Pause, Process and Progress.**

1. **Pause:** Work out when you can find some time and space to be with yourself and your feelings or you may decide to explore your feelings and trial these techniques with the support of a professional support or trusted friend or partner.

2. **Process:** Feel all the emotions you can identify, if feeling your feelings is either too uncomfortable or simply not possible for you, trial naming the emotion you might know is likely appropriate to the situation and move with that understanding of what you might be feeling, without experiencing the emotion directly. For example, you work out that the situation you are in could cause anger, you might then go for a fast-paced walk, run, hop on the spot or dance thinking about the feeling of anger. Make a connection with your body and your breath and see if you can feel any tension, then move with that tension until it starts to dissipate.

3. **Progress:** Once you sense your body and mind feel more at ease and the emotion, if you are feeling it, is less intense take a moment to reflect on the experience. Ask yourself questions that can help you ascertain if and how you could move forward from this experience into a space where you can make choices that may improve your situation or support your experience. Is there anything you might learn that could minimise or help you manage other similar emotional experiences? Are there

6. Positive Emotional Coping

are perceptions that could be altered or beliefs changed that might support creating different emotional experiences in the future? Were there any expectations that have beliefs underneath them that are not serving you well and could be altered with cognitive reprogramming and brain retraining?

Emotions are a natural and normal part of being human. Learning to support yourself through emotional experiences is a valid and worthwhile pursuit that may help make life feel more manageable, easeful, and safe. If none of the suggestions offered here resonate with you, consider continuing to explore other ideas or techniques that could assist you in identifying ways to manage emotions in a way that aligns with your values and does not lead to additional difficulties—either now or in the future.

Exercise: Developing Positive Emotional Management: Pause, Process, Progress

This exercise may help you trial the **Pause, Process and Progress** emotional management system using a previous experience to assess if it could be supportive for you. Focus on something small, nothing too intense or overwhelming, where you were upset but perhaps not devastated. This may allow you to see if this technique suits you, or if you can adapt it into something that might work better for you.

If you find this approach to emotional management supportive, you may choose to practice it regularly. Over time, repeated use of a helpful strategy may make it more familiar and accessible during times of emotional discomfort. With consistent reflection and application, your ability to respond to strong or uncomfortable feelings may gradually improve, supporting your overall wellbeing. Repetition can also help reinforce learning, which may contribute to more sustainable and adaptive emotional responses in the future.

Maybe consider taking this exercise to a professional therapist, counsellor, psychologist, or a trusted friend and work through the steps in a safe and supported environment. This is a deep reflective exercise that may not be appropriate to

6. Positive Emotional Coping

undertake without support, please consider use of this carefully in accordance with your own history and circumstances. We will provide two options to work with your feelings. One is very short, simple and appropriate to less intense emotional experiences and might be a gentler way to start using this practice. You are not likely to wish or be able to dive deeply into every single emotional experience and sometimes having a simpler tactic might be more fitting for yourself or the situation you are in.

Simpler Version:

Pick a recent emotional experience that left you feeling something uncomfortable such as anger, disappointment or sadness, nothing too intense or too big that might lead you to feeling overwhelmed. Then working with the following statements, say each one silently in your mind and focus in on the sensations you are feeling or observing in your body:

1. *I feel* ....

    Name the emotion if it is clear to you, if not simply focus on whatever it is you are feeling. Take a moment to be present with the sensations.

2. *I acknowledge* ....

    You might put the emotion to a situation, e.g. "I acknowledge that I feel angry at my partner" or just "I acknowledge that something is not feeling comfortable or right" and take another moment to be with whatever you feel. Feeling into and allowing the sensations to continue.

3. *I release* ....

   Let go of the feeling, the situation, or anything that feels appropriate to you in this moment to let go of. Stay with the moment if you can until the feeling of intensity has either subsided or disappeared.

More In-depth Version:

This is a much lengthier and more involved version. Consider undertaking this one perhaps after using the first tool for a while or with a therapist or trusted person to begin with whilst you learn how it might work for you.

Think of a recent example of when you became emotional, something that stirred up moderately intense feelings or provoked an emotional reaction from you. Then answer the questions below. An example of how to work with this process is given below.

Pause:

1. **Take a breath and be present. What is it I am feeling? (Identifying feelings and 'sub' feelings.)**

   Example – I tried to talk my partner about supporting my goals and they didn't seem to listen or care. This made me feel frustrated, dismissed and not important, especially as I always actively support their goals. It makes me feel lonely and not worthy.

2. **Where do these feelings come from, is it just about this one moment? Are there ideas I have been given about this situation that influence how I feel about it?**

6. Positive Emotional Coping

Example – I have felt this way before with my partner, they often get tangled up in their stuff and then have no space left for me. But is goes further back than that. My last partner also made me feel unimportant and I never felt my family got me either. I always admired the type of relationships where people supported each other in everything they did. This kind of mutual support is a value of mine and is important for me to feel safe and content.

3. **How do I get in my own way? Where is my responsibility in this?**

   Example – I have noticed that I can react strongly as past hurts get activated and this can impact my judgment of the present situation and can stop me from communicating clearly, I can forget my words. My partner has said that at times they feel blamed for all my bad experiences. I have some self-doubt and sometimes I need other people to help me feel better about myself because of this. I don't always back myself enough or encourage myself much, I can be very negative towards myself in my own mind. When I only rely on my partner making me feel good, I am risking a negative outcome, because when they cannot provide this, I feel bad, I wonder if I may to better off relying more on myself to feel confident and capable?

Process:

4. **Can I make some time to sit with my feelings first, before I communicate my needs? Is there anything from stopping me doing this?**

Example – I have not had time to sit with my feelings, I have a lot of other responsibilities, and I can easily forget about taking care of me. I notice that I get this urgency to get my feelings out to someone else, as that feels easier than sitting with them by myself and I think it could sort things out quicker. This is not always true though, and can make things worse when I rush in. I think it's important I sit with which feelings are relevant to my partner now to help improve the current situation, and I focus on letting go of the hurt from the past that I cannot change, and support myself more actively.

5. **Is there a fear here? Is that fear about the now, the past or the future? Can I manage my own fears? Are my fears absolute or relative truths?**

    Example – I fear not being taken seriously, not being heard. I fear that I will have to do things the way everyone else wants and my needs will not matter. I fear being blamed. I fear things won't change. These are all relative fears, relating back to past negative experiences. All these fears are things that I could maybe influence and possibly change, either by changing my mindset about myself or by changing the people who surround me and finding those who are more supportive.

6. **What can I let go of here? Is there a pattern here that if repeated might cause harm? Or is this something in 5 years' time I won't remember?**

    Example – It could help to let go of my past hurts from old partners and my family, and accept they were not able to support me in the way that I needed. I do not think this is a helpful pattern we are in where my partner gets so lost in their stuff it is to my detriment. I also think

6. Positive Emotional Coping

I could support myself more and be less reliant on others to believe I can achieve my goals. If my partner cannot create better space for me and I cannot support myself more, then our relationship may not last. I would like to help myself and address the issue with my partner, otherwise I could just repeat the pattern with someone else.

Progress:

7. **Can I learn from this and/or change my perspective to feel safer? Is this something I just have to accept or are there ways to work with people to create change?**

    Example – I have learned I really value positive support, and it is important for me in my intimate relationships. I can be kinder and more encouraging towards myself. I could look at the bigger picture of my relationship and see if they cannot provide this kind of support, do they meet all my other needs? I might ask myself, is the relationship good, apart from this one aspect that makes it worth accepting emotional support is not their skill? Or there are other issues that indicate this is not a good fit for me? Is there any risk or danger from staying in this relationship?

8. **Is there anyone I could communicate with to help me move forward? What is the most balanced approach I can take to express myself, and create clear communication to secure a better outcome for everyone?**

    Example – I can find a way to communicate with my partner about the feelings they evoke when they treat me a certain way. I can acknowledge some of these feelings are from my past. I can remind myself I am not back in the past to keep myself calm and be able to think clearly and put in boundaries with my partner if they talk over me. I can ask my partner to be present with me rather than diverting into blame or distraction. I can recognise the ways my partner makes me feel good. I can ask for their support in altering some of the ways they treat me, to help me feel heard and so we can both feel content and safe. If my partner is unwilling to work with me, I may consider how healthy this relationship is for me, and if being with someone who cannot be accountable, or help me feel safe to speak up and work with me on solutions is viable on the long-term.

9. **What else might help me during this difficult time and moving forward?**

    Example – I function better when I sleep or rest well, eat regularly and movement helps me think. I can talk to my trusted friends or see a therapist. Going out for some fun or playing games helps me have a break from the heavy stuff of processing emotions. Dropping into roles that have nothing to do with the situation also may help, especially those roles I know I do well in, like certain aspects of my job, being creative or being active and exercising. When I am in that more confident version of my identity, it can support the parts of me that feel afraid or doubtful.

If you find this exercise brings up difficult emotions, please pause and consider seeking support from a therapist or mental health professional.

6. Positive Emotional Coping

Pause — Reflect — Landscape

1. **Pause** - Take a moment to sit with what you have just learned and consider it.

- Without having an adaptable and sustainable positive emotional management system in place, we may find our ability to start and maintain change can be inhibited, limited or stopped.
- Building a positive emotional coping framework is supported by the skill of mindfulness.
- Mindfulness may assist us in assessing the present, checking the past and projecting into the future, to see what might happen if we follow the course of action our mind is considering.
- Being able to anchor into the present may allow us to hear our thoughts and potentially stop ourselves from doing something that could harm us or others.
- Emotions can be uncomfortable, but the intensity changes and they can pass, emotions may also help guide us towards making changes within ourselves and our lives.

- Assessing that our feelings are fair and valid allows us to see if there is anything we can do to support changing them by taking actions or reframing how we see the situation or how we see ourselves.

- Having a positive way to manage our emotions might help us feel it is possible to regain control, influence the direction we are moving in and create alternate outcomes.

- Knowing what might block us when dealing with our feelings could help create a clearer path and in making space to manage our feelings.

- Being solution-focused, and using self-compassion, encouragement and supporting ourselves well forms part of a positive emotional management framework.

- Learning to pause and identity our feelings, means we may then be able to process them, which could occur through letting ourselves feel our feelings or conscious movement, and we may then progress forwards with new information and knowledge that could help us cope with other future emotional experiences.

2. **Reflect** - Answer the following questions:

    - Are you someone who is comfortable to work with their feelings?
    - How do you normally deal with your feelings? Do you talk about them? Ignore them? Suppress them? Put them into some kind of activity or movement or another form of distraction?

6. Positive Emotional Coping

- Do you easily move into a state of overwhelm? Or feel like there is no more space left for you to hold any other feelings?

3. **Landscape** - Step back from the details and see how this new information fits in with the bigger picture of your life. Consider your history, what is going on for you now, who and what is in your life, and the future you want for yourself.

- ✓ Are there times in your life where you can see that your emotions or your experience of them got in the way of change? Do you think you would benefit from improving your emotional management system? What emotional management approaches that you currently use or have previously used work for you?

- ✓ Do you ever find when you get upset about something your emotional reaction is more intense than the situation would indicate, or is more than you expected? Are you holding pain from the past that is inflaming new emotional experiences and requires your attention or professional support?

- ✓ Who or what in your life could help you manage your emotions? Are you a very private person that prefers to work through things alone and does this always work well? Are there particular people in your life that can provide emotional support or is this kind of support something you could cultivate through building intimacy with others you trust? Can you identify any blocks to engaging with your feelings? these could come from experiences, attitudes or a belief that dealing with your feelings doesn't matter.

7. When Thinking Can be Bad for Your Health

In this section you will be learning about:

- → Why do we overthink?
- → What are the risks of negative overthinking?
- → How might we release ourselves from unhelpful overthinking loops?

You will need:

- ✓ A space to meditate.
- ✓ To be courageous when sitting in an uncomfortable experience.
- ✓ To remember that feelings are temporary.
- ✓ To make notes on any insights that arise.
- ✓ To be open to discussing your reactions, feelings, and ideas, either with yourself or others.

7. When Thinking Can be Bad for Your Health

"Overthinking is like being stuck on a hamster wheel, always moving but never advancing. "

Gael MacLean

Thinking can be bad for your health, at least it can be when you are overthinking and hyper-focusing on negatives. If you are busy overthinking, you might not be focusing or present, and when your overthinking is profoundly negative your confidence could naturally drop and this can affect your awareness of anything that may need changing or how you are managing the process of change. People often complain that they are overthinkers. Overthinking can be part of the joy of being human or a curse, depending on your point of view. What matters about thinking is not so much the amount we are thinking, but the **direction of our thinking**. When we get caught going down rabbit holes of reactivity, we may spiral through thoughts that are solely generated from a negative self-perspective. They might not be from an external, independent observer point of view and not always based on fact, sometimes they are fictional. They could be derived from either previous experiences or fears of the future or uncertainties about who we are. Once we start thinking about a negative event or experience, that feeling can attach to another similar thought or memory, and another, and another, and before we know it, we are stuck in some kind of negative freefall.

Obstacles that can get in the way of change and can lead to negative overthinking include having low self-worth that may not allow us to experience valid, positive feelings, like happiness at receiving a gift or pride at achieving something. For some, family history may predispose us to behaving in similar ways as our parents or grandparents, who may not have talked about their feelings or celebrated their wins. Our culture may lower our self-worth, where we are made to feel we are not equal to others or just not good enough and we should always be doing more, being more and having more. When we start understanding and recognising how these types of issues are playing out in our own internal conversations, we can start to consider new narratives. By challenging ideas of how we view ourselves and identifying what are the threats and the opportunities in any given situation, we can create a freedom of thought that allows us to feel very differently. In these ways we may start to manage any negative overthinking and potentially avoid the rabbit holes, and then any excessive thinking might become uplifting, motivating and supportive.

Science tells us we have around 12,000 thoughts a day. As much of our thinking is done via the subconscious/automatic mind, we are, in theory, not consciously aware of the vast majority of these thoughts. But some days it just doesn't feel that way. Some days, it feels like our heads might even implode from the amount of thinking we are doing. When we are immersed in this overthinking modality, we are typically very much not present in the moment, meaning we can be separated from potentially beautiful, important or fun experiences. Overthinking can

7. When Thinking Can be Bad for Your Health

definitely mar the moment. One of the most common complications arising from overthinking is our natural tendency to fill in the blanks. What this means is that, when we do not have all the information about a situation or we do not know exactly what someone is feeling or doing, we can start to add to the story, without having access to facts or actual knowledge. This is particularly unhelpful when that narrative is on the negative side of things. This can lead to us creating problems that might not exist, and having associated feelings that may be unnecessary as the situation in our mind is not actually happening or likely to ever happen.

A classic example of this might be if you have had the experience of someone cheating on you in a prior relationship. Because of the hurt and pain coming from this, you understandably want to avoid repeating the experience again. So, when, one day, your new partner comes home from work talking about their fabulous new colleague and how great they are, you start to feel uncomfortable, unsure if this means your new partner may have a romantic interest in this person. You avoid asking your partner about their feelings and continue to think about the situation. Any time your partner mentions this person's name, you wonder if they spend lunchtimes together or if they plan to be together at the office Christmas party. You then start to imagine them working late together and starting an affair. You forget to ask yourself along way the way, if what you are thinking about is a relative truth or an absolute truth. By this point, you could be feeling dreadful as you keep repeating this negative story to yourself about your new partner cheating on you, even though there is no evidence that this is the case. Your fear and overthinking have created a fictional story that has led you to feel horrible, and possibly resentful to a partner who may have done nothing wrong. This can lead to real conflict, hurting your partner, and even breaking up.

Imagine things going differently. From the first time you have suspicions, and regularly over time, the two of you openly and honestly share your feelings and talk about what is really going on. Doing this presents an opportunity to understand each other better and build greater trust than ever. Rather than hurt the relationship, the potential threat and your decision to tackle it as a team reinforces bonds and leads to a possibly brighter future. Instead of filling in the blanks, you are getting real time information. This is not to indicate we should ignore our suspicions or intuition and assume it is wrong. Sometimes our suspicions might turn out to be true even if we have talked about things openly. What this example shows us is that directly communicating with your partner is potentially more helpful than filling in the blanks yourself, as it removes unhelpful overthinking and the stress that can bring. We can then use our analytical thinking mind not from a space of fear, but from a place of **information seeking** and **solution finding**. Whether or not our partner really was cheating, directly confronting the issue is likely less painful and more productive than privately and endlessly stewing over what-ifs.

Negative overthinking becomes more dangerous the more you repeat thinking about something. As neuroscience tells us, the more we repeat a thought, the more likely we are to reinforce a negative belief and create a neural pathway to correspond to that negative belief so that it might remain in our brain. Finding ways to communicate with others, as well as showing yourself compassion and redirecting your thoughts to be more supportive can help prevent this negative programming.

Sometimes, despite having good communication or

7. When Thinking Can be Bad for Your Health

receiving accurate information that is supposed to be making us feel better and calmer, our minds can remain locked in the overthinking mode and cycle back to the negative. Here is some sage, old advice that may help the overthinker: it is better to laugh than cry. If you have been able to speak to your partner and they have allayed your fears, or you have resolved whatever situation you were overthinking, but those negative and fearful thoughts still continue, maybe you can find a gentle and kind way to laugh at yourself, perhaps with a healthy dose of compassion. Maybe you can admire your creativity and your imagination. Perhaps you can make light of your overthinking with others to diffuse and derail the overthinking mind. It is very much harder to feel sad or angry when laughter is filling your whole body. Instead of writing a tragedy in your mind, maybe you could put that imagination and overthinking to better use and write a fun and fulfilling success story in your head. Turn a negative behaviour into a positive one using your own talent for creativity to help you rather than harm you. An active imagination can be an advantage, and if you have addressed the issues you have been fearing, it may support the mind into a more positive paradigm. You can also turn to your strengths to help you out of the deluge of overthinking. What about focusing on your positives? How you treat others? The good things you do or have achieved? This may help you loosen the overthinking chains and bring yourself out of those negative spirals that are not leading to resolution, and instead spiralling endlessly inwards. Remember, it is not so much the overthinking that is the problem, but the direction of your thinking. If you are **overthinking positively**, you cannot help but feel positive.

Feeling guilty may also lead us into overthinking, along with hindsight bias. "We should have known better" is an argument no one can ever win because one cannot infallibly predict outcomes. We can become stuck in rumination, procrastination, and even ambivalence if we do not manage our overthinking minds more positively. You can use the absolute and relative truth equation to help you find your original intention in amongst the guilty thoughts, did you intend to cause harm or end up with this particular outcome? There might be occasions that we would do better to get out of the overthinking mode and be better off to get into our feelings. At times, overthinking may start with a feeling like fear, worry, paranoia, anxiety, disappointment, or guilt. Whatever the emotion is, we may try to avoid feeling the emotion by overthinking about it and then create other feelings to be managed, without any of them necessarily being required. In such moments sometimes, the way out of our heads is to feel our feelings, without engaging the thinking brain, simply acknowledging them and allowing them to exist and then releasing them. This might not be comfortable, but at least you are only dealing with the initial feelings rather than all the others created from overthinking and fictional filling-in of the blanks. This also might give you a better platform from which to engage in solutions that could help you from repeating the overthinking, such as talking things over and seeking out more information or finding something to make you laugh.

Remember to get to the flow state or in the zone, where we can really excel, we cannot go from the negative mind to the no mind. We first become **accomplished at the positive** mind. If you have a talent for overthinking, change the direction of your thoughts to be positive, uplifting, nurturing, and supportive. The outcome may pleasantly surprise you. It might not be that less is more here, but maybe it is quality and quantity.

Exercise: Sitting with Pain Meditation

A way out of overthinking could be to sit and feel your feelings. It's not necessarily pleasant or easy to do, but it could be an opportunity to change the pattern. We can become so adept at dissociating from our feelings and be so out of our body and stuck in the rabbit warren of self-defeatism that we may completely convince ourselves that we do not feel anything and cannot do anything. Or we may just feel so plain terrified of feeling our feelings that we cannot even start the process.

Learning to sit with our feelings, practicing holding them and then releasing them is challenging. But it can be a healing process that may allow us to soften the experience of uncomfortable emotions by letting them be felt and then released. Feelings do lessen, things can change.

Maybe consider taking this exercise to a professional therapist, counsellor, psychologist, or a trusted friend and work through the steps in a safe and supported environment. This is a deep reflective exercise that may not be appropriate to undertake without support, please consider use of this carefully in accordance with your own history and circumstances.

This exercise is available on our website to listen to. You may wish to use this exercise as a way to gently begin practicing how to sit with your emotions until they naturally shift or ease. It can be helpful to start with a mild or manageable emotion rather than something deeply distressing. Over time, as you feel more confident, you might gradually explore more challenging emotional experiences. Repeating this practice consistently may support the development of emotional awareness and resilience.

- Sit quietly, breathing deeply, and draw your awareness to your breath.
- Allow yourself to lean in toward your breath, perhaps with a soft feeling of curiosity.
- Once you feel settled, shift your focus to your body and look for any places in the body where you are holding emotional or physical pain. Lean gently towards this area and feeling, if you can, go carefully, deeper into it. Lean back out if it feels too much and return to the breath.
- If and when you feel ready, bring your focus fully to that area. You may be able to identify the emotion (e.g., anger, fear, anxiety).
- Do not think about why you are feeling this emotion.
- Do not try to talk yourself out of feeling it or judge it.
- Do not try to ignore your feeling or distract yourself.
- Instead, focus on feeling it and simply breathe through it until it begins to subside. Allow yourself to face the emotion, allowing it to exist and then dissipate, without thinking about what's behind it.
- Continue until either the pain or feeling has gone, and you can ease out of it. Or hold this space for 5 to 20 minutes, or until it becomes too much.

7. When Thinking Can be Bad for Your Health

- Repeat as required (you may need to go over the same areas or feeling many times).

If you find this exercise brings up difficult emotions, please pause and consider seeking support from a therapist or mental health professional.

Exercise: Playing with Time

There are times we want to hang onto good feelings and make them last as long as possible. Then, there are times we want to a moment to pass as quickly as possible. Negative overthinking can get in the way of good times and it can become out of control when we are stressed or worried about something or waiting impatiently for that good thing to come. We might be waiting for a special friend to visit, and we are excited, or we may have to see the dentist and feel scared and uncomfortable. There are many situations where we might wish we could control time because the feeling is either comfortable or uncomfortable. Whilst time cannot be controlled, we may at times be able to alter our perception of time, and we can achieve this through positive presence. Overthinking can be useful for achieving this.

The two exercises below provide you with steps to take to either make a moment last or to make it go by quicker. Use both and see if you can train yourself into using them mindfully whenever you might wish to speed things up or slow things down.

A word of warning

Do not play with time to speed up the bad things that are better off being felt and dealt with, or for slowing down the good things to avoid getting to problems that may need resolving. This is a tool that can be overused, so be careful when implementing it. Use these strategies carefully. They are to be used selectively. Otherwise, if you keep speeding time up to get to the good parts, you are not going to properly process uncomfortable feelings. This tool then becomes another form of denial or avoidance, both of which are unhealthy and not sustainable. Before using these techniques, take a moment to consider if you are playing with time in a healthy manner or using it to circumvent doing the emotional work that might need to be done.

Slowing Time Down

To slow time down, we can become incredibly present. By being connected to the moment through all our senses, we can absorb ourselves completely in whatever is going on. There are no thoughts about the future and what is coming next. There are no thoughts about the past and what has happened before. This overthinking is all done in the present moment. Don't time slip into the past or the future as this could lead to creating other issues that are either unhelpful or irrelevant.

We pay attention to all the small details. What can you hear? What can you see? What can you smell? What can you feel? What can you sense or touch? Are there are tastes? Ease into each one of the senses, taking note of everything you recognise. Keep coming back to the senses to ground you in every single moment, taking in as much as you can about it without letting the mind go forward or backward in time. Fully immerse in the moment mentally, emotional, physically and creatively.

Speeding Time Up

If the art of slowing time down comes from being hyper-present, the art of speeding time up comes from being as absent as possible from the present moment. Do not use this technique when driving or operating machinery, or during anything that requires your presence and focus for safety.

Allow your mind to wander to things you might be looking forward to. Or stretch your mind back to moments in the past that were beautiful and fun. Dive into the details of your time travel. What can you remember from that past moment? What did you feel? What was said? What was the weather like? Or what do you hope will happen in the future? What are you going to feel? What order might things happen in? Who might be there? What might they say? Be somewhere else in your mind and the present might feel like it is slipping away seemingly quicker. Literally, overthink every positive detail.

Reminder!

If you are speeding time up to get to the next good moment, be sure to consciously slow time back down again, as your mind might be stuck in the gear set for racing through time, and you could miss the very thing you have been looking forward to.

Also be wary of setting high expectations that might not get met. Just because you imagined an event happening one way, be aware it could play out very differently, and that's OK. Flow with the experience, and do not judge it against your imagination unfairly.

If you find this exercise brings up difficult emotions, please pause and consider seeking support from a therapist or mental health professional.

7. When Thinking Can be Bad for Your Health

Pause—Reflect—Landscape

1. **Pause** - Take a moment to sit with what you have just learned and consider it.

- Overthinking is less of an issue than the direction of your thinking, i.e. is it positive or negative? Negative overthinking may create stress. Positive overthinking may generate energy and motivation.
- Negative overthinking can affect and block change when it is not managed.
- Low self-worth from our experiences, relationships and the media can encourage negative overthinking, spiralling us down into reactive rabbit holes that can lead us from one difficult thought to another, maybe accumulating to make us feel we are not good enough, there is no way out, or we are not capable.
- We might avoid the rabbit warrens of negative overthinking by challenging ourselves to think more kindly and positively.
- Filling in the blanks with unverified information feeds negative overthinking and can make us feel anxious, depressed and vulnerable

- Seeking out further information, developing open communication with others and checking if we are working with absolute truths or relative truths, could ameliorate and reduce negative overthinking.

- Repetitive negative overthinking can build neural pathways, setting us up for automatic negative thoughts that can harm us again, and again.

- Feeling our feelings can reduce negative overthinking and playing with time can aid us in putting overthinking to good use.

- Laughter may diffuse and minimise the impacts of negative overthinking and could derail unhelpful trains of thoughts or stop us from filling in the blanks with unhelpful information.

- We can actively change negative overthinking into a positive direction using our imagination, our strengths and successes to create a different story.

2. **Reflect** - Answer the following questions:

   - Have you noticed any situations or subjects where you are thinking a lot? Do you worry about the future? Or create scripts or write stories in your head based only on a few facts? Do you ruminate on negative past events that you cannot change?

   - What kinds of feelings do you experience when you are thinking excessively? Does the overthinking have any other consequences, can you become irritable, stressed or even paranoid?

7. When Thinking Can be Bad for Your Health

3. **Landscape** - Step back from the details and see how this new information fits in with the bigger picture of your life. Consider your history, what is going on for you now, who and what is in your life, and the future you want for yourself.

- ✓ Are you able to see any periods of your life or situations where overthinking negatively either distracted you from addressing things that needed to be changed or affected you sustaining changes you were in the process of making? Can you see how the overthinking affected you? What might you be able to address in this pattern of behaviour around your overthinking?

- ✓ Do you know why you overthink? Are you naturally analytical? Are you very creative? Have your bad experiences led you to seek control by preparing for every eventuality? Does your overthinking stem from feeling anxious or believing you are not good enough?

- ✓ What strengths can you use to manage overthinking, your creativity, asking friends for help, better communication with others? Could you use humour to manage out of control thinking? If you do not manage your overthinking better, what might happen?

8. Attachment – The Sticky Tape of the Mind

In this section you will be learning about:

- → Why do we develop and maintain attachments?
- → How can we misunderstand attachment and misjudge letting go?
- → What stops us from letting go?
- → How can we free ourselves from unhelpful attachments in a healthy way?

You will need:

- ✓ Time to reflect.
- ✓ A willingness to see what may hold you back from letting go at times.
- ✓ An attitude of preparedness to confront yourself.
- ✓ To be open to discussing your reactions, feelings, and ideas, either with yourself or others.

8. Attachment – The Sticky Tape of the Mind

Self-awareness is the ability to take an honest look at your life without any attachment to it being right or wrong, good or bad.

Debbie Ford

Some common advice offered to those in emotional distress or discomfort is to let it go. This might occur, for example, after you have expressed a frustration about your workplace, something that you cannot influence or change and the person you are telling about it simply says you need to let it go. Another example might relate to receiving some negative feedback from someone whose opinion matters to you, and you are stuck ruminating on it and again people advise you to let it go. It could refer to a relationship you thought was going to last that has ended and you felt like this was the only person for you and you are unable to let go of your feelings or release the hope you might get back together, or the relationship has become toxic and unhealthy, but you can't seem to walk away. There are many situations in our lives where letting go seems to be the favoured advice but achieving the letting go can be a lot harder or more complex. When we cannot let go, we cannot change things completely or fully.

Unhelpful attachment occurs when we are hanging onto feelings that may not serve us, or we are sticking with ideas or ideals that no longer suit our circumstance, or we are holding onto an outcome that is no longer possible or staying in a situation that is not tenable. Mastering the art of letting go or detachment doesn't mean you won't feel emotions. You may still need to process grief, loss, and the many other feelings that arise along the way. Letting go is not about denying your feelings but instead the adjustment of an attitude or a belief to help you process the feelings and move forward from the experience that has caused disappointment, distress or discomfort.

Attachment implies that there is a need that can only be fulfilled by hanging on to whatever it is that we are attached to. If we become attached, we may become entrapped and stuck in something that is not supportive or helpful to us. Attachment may not allow us to process our feelings fully, and thus, potentially be freer to move forward onto something new that could help us grow and change or even find something that makes us happier. We can struggle with attachment because it is often very densely emotional. Detaching or letting go is a hard one to suss out, so please do not let your mind lurch into negative judgment over whether you attach or cannot detach. It's a tough skill to develop, but one that may come with mindful care and attention and could bring both relief and opportunity with it.

Attachment and our ego can at times have an intimate relationship. The idea that we must have something could come from a fear that we are less without it, incomplete, or unable to do anything. These are relative to your beliefs, not necessarily based on facts that you cannot be without whatever it is you are attached to. This is likely a fear-driven concept, shaped more by personal belief than by absolute truth. It is often a supposition born of anxiety. The fear of lacking something in life can arise directly from the ego. Awareness

8. Attachment – The Sticky Tape of the Mind

can support us in navigating into a place of being content as things are. It may help us to recognise that we have whatever we need in the moment or helps us prepare to take positive action to find what would be required to make the best of a situation, all couched within an active embrace of patience and acceptance. This can help reduce feelings of dependency, dismantle attachments to specific outcomes, and create a sense of timeliness, where there is less rush to have it all now or hold onto it forever.

Being attached to an outcome can be a source of pain and frustration. When we set goals, we rarely think to set an intention or plan for what happens if we cannot achieve or meet this goal. Yet this kind of thinking can be progressive, preparatorily helpful, and could help us respond more calmly to change. It may not feel easy or comfortable to do and we could fear it might mean we are being negative. But focusing on an alternate outcome, or being aware things might not work out as hoped, is not about being resigned to inevitable failure nor need it adversely affect your confidence. But **supporting your future self** by thinking about all possible outcomes could be beneficial in the long run. For example, a woman deeply wants a child and goes to great lengths to have one, only to find she cannot get pregnant. She is devastated, sad, and feels lost without the chance to have her own children. By being prepared for another outcome from the outset, there is a chance that she may have a different, softer and less intensely painful experience. She may find it easier to accept that this might not be her path and recognise that there could be other ways that she can have an experience of being a parent. Or she could find other ways to enjoy life and create connections that could be just as satisfying for her. Therefore, should she not get pregnant, whilst she would understandably still be very sad, disappointed and need to grieve this outcome, there would be the hope of other joys there, waiting in the wings. This method of detachment to outcomes does not stop you having any feelings, nor would it stop the same feelings returning at other times in your life. You may still have to sit with the loss and sadness when something you want does not eventuate and manage this over time. But it creates an alternative pathway forward should it be needed and provides the mind with another positive way to resolve those feelings, potentially more expediently. No one is saying don't be positive or hopeful, just be ready to embrace an adaptation to the plan if it is required.

Being able to detach does not mean that you never fall in love and always keep people at a distance. It does not mean that you do not grieve the person who is no longer with you. Detaching from the career you longed for and trained for does not mean it wasn't important to you or make the loss of a passion easy. It means that you don't hang onto the perception that this one person, this one thing, or this one role was the only chance you had to be happy or complete. Using your expectations exercise from Book, 1 you can see if you have some unhelpful beliefs underneath any unwillingness to let something go or any blocks to being positive or peaceful about alternate outcomes that could eventuate.

When we are fixating on possessing and having something or someone, tomorrow and the next day and the next, we can be solely focused on a future that does not exist and that we cannot completely control. This may put us out of present time and might mean we are not fully available to the moment or loving the person we are with or situation we are in, we could become immersed in thinking about how we can keep

8. Attachment – The Sticky Tape of the Mind

this thing we are fixated on needing it or having it to be ok. This could put us at risk from either disappointment when we cannot maintain the status quo or trying to control things and possibly disregard the needs of others. When today is enough, it can also support the idea that you are enough, because you are not weighed down or dependent on the need, you are free you enjoy what is. This may give you a feeling of wholeness and completion, a comfortable emotional experience. It may allow you to accept that it might not always be there, but you are glad to have it whilst you do.

When we learn to let go, it does not mean that we never had those feelings or do not honour them by still feeling them. It means we have recognised that whatever purpose that relationship, role, or thing provided, it is no longer possible or able to be explored. There might be sadness, but sadness can be beautiful as it represents a recognition of love and joy. When there is **no attachment to an outcome,** then we may reduce the risk of misery. Misery is far from beauty; misery is suffering and hard. When we release a specific outcome, we may find the eventual outcome can change us in ways we could not foresee but be ok that it did, without having had the intense misery part as we were able to let go of what we loved, wanted, hoped for, or worked so hard for, accepting we could find a way to be ok without it.

Overthinking in negative circles encourages and supports attachment. Being a directional thinker means you can move forward. **Reflective thinking** can be a useful tool when it comes to managing our wellbeing and safety, it may allow us to look at what has worked well, what didn't and help us to adjust our approach in the future. Reflexive thinking differs in that the assessment of what is working and what isn't occurs in real time. This can make it a much more transformational process, taking our level of understanding of how we are helping or hindering ourselves much deeper. The **reflexive thinker is more self-aware**, using mindfulness at a high level to assess the situation as it unfolds and changing course accordingly, accessing their ability to look at why things are the way that they are and consider the role they are playing in the current moment and the potential outcome. So, while the reflective thinker analyses what has happened, the reflexive thinker automatically self-assesses and reacts to the circumstances as they are happening from a place of deeper self-understanding. They know themselves well and look inwardly as well as outwardly in order to create the best possible outcomes for all involved.

When thinking reflexively there is a level of responsibility that doesn't get reached with reflective practice alone. A reflexive thinker not only reflects on their own mind and what they know of how their mind can work, they think about the situation they are in and the people involved. They direct their thoughts rather than allow them to cascade into one another and start spiralling into emotional overwhelm and emotional reactivity. They choose their thoughts to move in a more appropriate direction. They find a balance between understanding that some events pertain to the actions of others, and some to the actions of themselves. They have greater psycho-diversity and this gives them access to a selection of positive coping skills. They can adapt from thinking about themselves, to others, to the situation, to previous experiences, and utilise all this information to aid in their decision-making and coping in the moment. They know when they can let go and when to hold a boundary. **Being a reflexive thinker can make letting go of attachments an easier process**, and instead of

8. Attachment – The Sticky Tape of the Mind

potentially holding on for longer than is good for you, you can detach and realign into a new direction sooner. This potentially saves you time, energy and emotional resources that can be depleted from hanging on or remaining stuck when attached.

For example, you are at work and your manager is unhappy with your performance and they start to have a go at you. Their anger and disappointment starts to feel like it is overwhelming you because your manager is clearly heightened and not in control of their own emotional regulation. As a reflexive thinker, you recall that your employer is under significant stress with the current restructure, and they confided in you the other day their marriage is also under strain. Remembering this and correlating it with the current moment allows you to take a mental and energetic step backwards from their tirade with some clear recognition their frustrations are not just about you and your performance, and not all your responsibility. You can also recognise that you too have been under a lot of strain and been given more work than you can manage during work hours, so you have been working late without being paid. You know you like your job and cannot afford to lose it, so this means you need to find a diplomatic way to now manage your manager. Once your manager feels seen and validated, they may calm themselves down, this allows you then you to take steps together to address the larger issue in a caring, but clear way, asserting your boundaries that you are already doing too much and that perhaps together you can find solutions to the issues. In doing so, you are protecting your current self and your role, possibly protecting your future self from taking on too much extra work, and protecting your relationship with your manager, and maybe even protecting your manager from themselves.

Tips for Becoming a Reflexive Thinker

This is high-level skill to learn, it requires the ability to not only remain present, but to know yourself well and be able to transition into the past to see what influences from your experiences might be activated in the situation and combine this knowledge with what you know about the other people involved, transition to the future to see where certain courses of action could end up, all whilst maintaining self-awareness and using self-knowledge and be able to sidestep emotional reactivity and remain calm and in control.

When learning to be more reflexive in our thinking, we have to be careful not to spiral into anxiety, big emotional responses or move into overthinking or try to micromanage every tiny aspect. To help avoid this trap we can support a balanced approach by using our intuition with our knowledge. Intuition is described as having the ability to know something instinctively without needing to engage conscious thinking, we all have access to this natural human ability, but we can improve our relationship with our intuition to also support reflexive thinking. By building comfort and confidence in our abilities, reading our body's reactions and practicing feeling into situations we may increase our trust in our instinctual capabilities.

Ultimately, this is a type of thinking that takes a great deal of practice and requires you to learn the individual components well and then put them all together. But this kind of thinking could be transformative, making life and relationships potentially feel more manageable and supporting us to feel calmer, possibly safeguarding our future wellbeing and

8. Attachment – The Sticky Tape of the Mind

help us take better care of our relationships through compassionate, careful and informed decision-making.

Steps to Reflexivity

Here are some steps you can take to build up the individual skills that may lead to more reflexive ways of thinking over time. Once you feel confident using the individual skills you can start to consciously combine them in real-time to see if they help you manage situations more effectively. There is no need to doubt your mental capacity to conduct this type of thinking practice and operate so many functions at the same time. Both your conscious and subconscious minds are capable of processing significant amounts of information in a single second. Practicing and repeating these steps below consistently may support the development of reflexive thinking skills, where your mind can handle this level of complex real-time reflection, assessment, thinking and decision-making.

1. Look at what you know about yourself.
   - What things can activate you or affect your emotional wellbeing?
   - Are you prone to insecurity and needing validation from others?
   - What helps to calm you or reassure you?
   - What makes you feel more capable and confident, and how can you increase that feeling for yourself?
   - Are there things from the past that adversely affect you, that you need to be mindful of and manage?

   Get to know yourself as well as possible from a place of

compassion and being non-judgmental. Don't criticize yourself for anything, but support yourself to looking after those things that don't work so well or are a bit fragile.

2. Develop the ability to be able to acknowledge and sit with your feelings, breathe through them and release them.

   Practice detachment so you can be clear of emotional clutter that could negatively impact decision-making and protective planning for all possible outcomes.

3. Practice being present and listening in on what your mind is telling you to think, or do, or say, and learn to question it.
   - Is what your mind offering up an absolute truth or relative truth?
   - Is that truth helpful in this situation?

   Use breathwork, meditations and other exercises that help you fully witness the present moment, so it feels safe and more comfortable after a while to do so.

4. Practice being a reflective thinker. Become accustomed to analysing situations after they occur to see what worked, what didn't work and what could be changed next time. Once this feels comfortable, start to assess situations as they happen using the same questions to see what is working, what isn't and what could create a good outcome for everyone.

5. Above all, learn to trust in yourself that you can approach things fairly, without using bias to protect

8. Attachment – The Sticky Tape of the Mind

yourself from being accountable or avoiding difficult change, and remind yourself, all things do eventually pass, and you can get through even the most challenging of situations and still be comfortable to be you.

Exercise: Detachment of Attachment

This exercise may give you ideas and insights on how to be able to detach and let go by using the following steps. This exercise can be very challenging if you are facing major life changes. Be gentle, and do not rush into it, maybe consider starting off with letting go of a small hurt or disappointment or you might consider undertaking this exercise with a professional therapist or when receiving some informal support from someone you trust. This might be something that takes time, space and professional help, there may be profound reasons why letting go is very hard and challenging for you, honour this and choose compassionate actions that can support and nurture you, not force you into something you are not ready for yet.

Letting go is not a quick thing. It is an individual, gradual process that you can choose and direct as you need to. Do not negatively judge your attachment, be gentle, kind and compassionate towards yourself. Do this in your time, not according to the schedule of others. Softly and kindly work with it to move into a more adaptable and sustainable way of being.

1. Openly and gently acknowledge to yourself what you are trying to hang onto and why. Offer yourself compassion and non-judgment.

8. Attachment – The Sticky Tape of the Mind

2. Ask yourself with kindness to accept that you can still be yourself without this person/role/thing/outcome you are attached to. You can still be content and fulfilled. You can still find connection and purpose.

3. Guide yourself towards positive actions that can help shift your energy into that acceptance by being present, such as movement, yoga, walking mindfully or being creative. Make the most of the moment through engaging all your senses to increase the sensation of accepting the now.

4. Allow space to just be with the feeling of acceptance and acknowledging that this part of your life is complete. Perhaps making room for alternate options for your future to appear in your mind. Maybe you take some time listening to others and their ideas or suggestions and support yourself to not become fixated on any one new alternate outcome.

5. Look out for statements you have made to yourself or others that indicate the presence of an attachment and work on a different way of seeing that situation. Something you must have or need. Something that without you would feel lost or you could not be yourself. Find an openness to other possible outcomes and being ok with them.

6. Are there feelings you can process using positive emotional management instead of using attachment as a coping mechanism?

7. See if your ego is trying to express attachment in some way by seeking labels or validation such as being an

athlete, a policeman, a wife, or a father, making you feel you cannot be without these labels because you are afraid of what will or will not happen without them. Gently see if the ego believes there are no other options for you and ask if this is really true? Ask yourself what is the fear telling you? Maybe use your fear management protocol to help you and use the information to support yourself.

- Remain compassionate and be ok if this takes time and you need to ease yourself into letting go. This is not meant to be a once and done process, nor should it take only a few seconds. This entire process could take some time and it's ok if it does, move at your pace, just be aware of getting stuck, delaying unnecessarily and making sure that it is not so slow that it is causing you or others harm or putting you or others at risk.

If you find this exercise brings up difficult emotions, please pause and consider seeking support from a therapist or mental health professional.

8. Attachment – The Sticky Tape of the Mind

Pause — Reflect — Landscape

1. **Pause** - Take a moment to sit with what you have just learned and consider it.

- Attachment can be unhelpful when we hang onto something that no longer serves us. Attachment can limit and block change.

- Letting go or detaching doesn't mean that we don't experience uncomfortable feelings, but instead it may allow us to feel our feelings and creates space for something new once they pass.

- When we believe we need something or rely on a particular outcome to be ok, this could be coming out of the ego mind. We fear we are less or incomplete somehow or unable to be happy/successful/content without whatever it is we are attached to. This is a relative truth, dependent only on our perception of the circumstances and not an absolute truth. We cannot truly know that we can't survive or live a good life without whatever it is.

- We can use our expectations as a guide to underlying beliefs that are creating unhelpful or harmful attachments.

- Creating opportunities for alternate outcomes may help us let go more easily and re-orientate into positive spaces.

- Being present and enjoying the now and trusting in our ability to cope with change can aid with detachment, should it be necessary.

- Overthinking may support unhelpful attachments. Being a reflective thinker can allow us to step back and assess situations and then adjust to another outcome.

- Reflexive thinking may allow us to be mindful in the moment and adjust actions in real-time to create supportive outcomes for both ourselves and others, potentially making attachment easier to manage and prevent.

- To become a reflexive thinker, it may help to know ourselves well, be present and self-reflect, learn to witness others and recall what we know about them, listen to what our mind is telling us, sit with and manage our feelings and reactions, and practice witnessing and analysing situations to be able to identify adjustments that benefit others, as well as ourselves.

2. **Reflect** - Answer the following questions:

    - How do you think you handle letting things go? Is this easy for you? Do you tend to hang onto things for longer than is healthy for you?

    - What can get in your way of being able to detach from things that do not serve you?

8. Attachment – The Sticky Tape of the Mind

- Are you a reflective thinker? Is this something you could learn or evolve into the higher-level skill of reflexive thinking?

3. **Landscape** - Step back from the details and see how this new information fits in with the bigger picture of your life. Consider your history, what is going on for you now, who and what is in your life, and the future you want for yourself.

- ✓ When you look back over your life, has retaining any attachments, to ideas, values, people or situations affected your ability to action and complete the process of change? Do you have any current attachments that could create issues for you in the future if you do not prepare for alternate outcomes or possibilities?

- ✓ What might it mean for how you live your life and cope with problems or stress if you were to become a more reflective or even reflexive thinker? What would be the direct benefits to you? Are there negative consequences if you don't adopt these skills?

- ✓ What can you use from what you have learned so far about yourself to become a reflexive thinker? Have the insights into you shown any opportunities or threats to being reflexive in your thinking? Any blocks you might need to overcome first?

9. Review of Insights into You

There are a number of internal and external challenges that may compromise and affect our capacity to change; by becoming more aware of their propensity to become obstacles to our growth we can identify and address them using adaptive tools and tactics to support us towards our goals, whilst aligning with our core values. During this Book we've discussed how the neuroplastic nature of the brain may support change and adaptation over time. Rather than having a set mind that assumes we cannot grow or evolve, we may begin to cultivate a more flexible perspective and mindset that allows us to develop new beliefs and habits through repeated practice. We have encouraged you to approach change with patience and compassionate care. Gradual repetition of new ways of thinking and behaving may help embed more adaptive habits that better serve our wellbeing. We may find that, over time, these practices become more accessible and less effortful, particularly when aligned with what we have chosen for ourselves, rather than being influenced by others.

We've explored the importance of acknowledging our complexity. We are beautifully complex; embrace it, be at peace with it and smile. Human behaviour and emotional patterns are rarely one-dimensional, and simplifying the process of change may overlook important factors. For example, creating a thought like "I'm confident in my job" might be more effective when paired with beliefs such as "I trust my ability to cope when things don't go to plan." Recognising the many roles and aspects that make up our identity may strengthen our sense of self and offer resilience in times of transition.

Awareness of cognitive tendencies like unconscious, hindsight and confirmation bias may also support clearer thinking. By practising self-reflection—such as moving into 'witness mode'—we might become better equipped to assess whether our thoughts are helpful or influenced by external pressures. In witness mode, we can assess information without the clutter of biases and identify if there might be factors we have not yet considered or observe if people may have their own agenda and are not necessarily acting in our best interests, potentially negatively affecting our conclusions or actions. This reflective approach can offer more balanced insights, helping us feel more grounded in our decisions.

Mindfulness and breathing techniques, like the ones introduced here, are simple strategies that may support this reflective process and being able to witness both ourselves and others. They can provide a moment of pause, allowing space for insight, redirection, and improved emotional regulation. By using breathing and witnessing exercises to help still the noise of the world and connect with ourselves, we can start to mine the mind for information regarding our beliefs and thoughts. This information can then be used to develop insights into what might be unhelpful or harmful and we may then create affirmations to retrain our brain into holding a different perspective or supporting ourselves more compassionately. These strategies are not quick fixes but may be valuable tools with regular practice, helping us stay focused and make thoughtful, values-aligned decisions.

We've considered ways to question unhelpful thought

9. Review of Insights into You

patterns by exploring whether they are based on absolute truths or relative truths, shaped by past experiences, people and perceptions. Our conscious mind may play a key role in identifying and reshaping these beliefs over time. Rather than relying solely on our mind for verbatim direction, we can learn to **question** where **our mind** is trying to take us, asking, does this way of thinking really help me? Is this coming from me or an unhelpful influence? Is it based on an absolute truth or a relative truth? Once answered, these questions can help guide us change course as necessary.

Coping techniques can be both helpful and harmful depending on the proportion with which we use them. Knowing this aids us in how we use them. Be mindful of overusing denial, diversion, distraction, and avoidance. They may only work sporadically and in the short term. If we deny something is happening to us, or a behaviour belongs to us, or avoid our feelings, then there is nothing we can do about it. Whilst a situation that was not our fault may have caused us harm; we may have to address how we have been hurt and how we might move forward from it. This is the part we can control and influence through compassionate approaches to mindful self-care. Returning to our personal strengths—such as our resilience, or our unwillingness to give up, courage, or creativity—can also support us during emotional challenges. By recognising our role in managing thoughts and responses, we may feel more empowered to shift from blame or avoidance to accountability and growth.

Difficult emotions like guilt or fear may influence our ability to process feelings and block or hamper our efforts to change. Creating a compassionate internal response to these emotions, while developing strategies to cope, may help us feel more emotionally supported. It can be helpful to work with frameworks that promote compassion and acceptance, especially during moments of reflection or difficulty. Using our intention as a guide to help us understand where our behaviour has come from can aid in showing ourselves kindness for what has occurred. We cannot change what was, but we can actively influence who we are and what is yet to come. In this way, we may be able to own it and grow from it.

Throughout this process we have encouraged you to view your emotions as signals, helpful indicators that something may need your attention. Accepting and validating our emotional experiences can support us in feeling our feelings, by whichever adaptive means suits us and this may then lead us into a place where we might either resolve, reduce or manage our emotional experiences with less intensity, less impact and more kindness. While some coping strategies offer relief in the short term (e.g., avoidance or distraction), they may not support long-term wellbeing and can affect the process of change, stalling it or preventing it. Exploring what helps us feel safe and grounded during emotional discomfort could be beneficial. Strategies like "pause, process, progress" can be adapted to suit our needs. Learning how to be more comfortable when we are emotionally uncomfortable can support healthy emotional management and facilitate our progress towards change.

Similarly, when faced with overthinking, we may consider whether our thought patterns are helping us move forward or keeping us stuck. Redirecting focus, connecting with others, and challenging limiting narratives can offer relief. Managing overthinking can be supported by ascertaining in which direction our thoughts are taking us. It may be more helpful to land in a positive and solution-focused train of thought, rather than

9. Review of Insights into You

ruminating on the negatives. We might be able to break out of negative overthinking by seeking out information through communicating with others, focusing on our strengths, feeling our feelings and letting them go or by being creative with the stories we are telling ourselves and turn them into brighter or even funnier ones to help shift the pattern and release any overwhelming emotion. Use your other skills, such as your imagination and your capacity to be curious to engage and drive overthinking rather than letting it overtake you.

Letting go of attachments, and especially attachments to singular outcomes, is another powerful skill. By reflecting on what we hope or anticipate from a situation, we may be able to soften the emotional impact if things don't go as we want them to or as expected. Flexibility can reduce the burden of disappointment and allow us to remain open to alternative outcomes, allowing change to evolve continuously in line with our circumstances. Being able to manage letting go and activating conscious detachment could be an assistive practice in managing uncomfortable emotions and facilitating change. By getting ahead of ourselves to identify what we think, or hope will happen, we may be able to support ourselves into accepting various possible outcomes and this may alleviate or reduce the possibility of prolonged emotional discomfort and feeling overwhelmed if things do not go as wished. Detaching from attachment can remove the blocks that could prevent us from discovering new opportunities that could be beneficial in ways that we could not foresee.

Learning the skills to become a reflexive thinker could be beneficial, when thinking reflexively we may be able to witnesses situations and ourselves in real-time and then consider information and actively manage our reactions and feelings, moving towards letting go of anything that may not serve us or others, and this may support us in making choices that offer a promising outcome for all involved. The reflexive thinker is developing an ongoing awareness of what's happening within them and around them and responding with intention, using their psychodiversity to support and guide them in managing and responding to any obstacles they come across.

When attempting any form of change we can benefit from creating a more supportive internal dialogue. Our thoughts can shape our emotional environment, and with practice, we might replace critical or limiting inner commentary with more affirming, constructive messages. This can help us maintain through the repetitive and potentially difficult or dull demands required for change to become integrated into our daily lives and stay the course to achieve our goals.

A kind and supportive inner dialogue, combined with a positive emotional coping framework, can assist in navigating guilt, managing fear, and using overthinking in constructive ways. The ability to let go of attachments to outcomes that are no longer available—creating space for new opportunities—alongside minimal reliance on unhelpful coping strategies, may help us respond more effectively to life's challenges. When we use emotions as signals for areas needing attention and apply both reflective and reflexive thinking to enhance our adaptability, we may be better equipped to support long-term change and personal growth. Ultimately, meaningful change often involves multiple layers, because human beings are multi-layered. You are not expected to master these concepts overnight. Take your time, be kind to yourself, and honour the process as you go.

9. Review of Insights into You

Exercise: Insights Gained into you

Go back over the exercises you have completed and the insights you have noted, then answer the following questions. The information gathered here may be useful when reading Book 3.

1. What is the difference between a set mind and mindset? Do you have more of a set mind than a mindset? Are there areas in your life you have a mindset but, in some areas, it is a set mind? Which of the techniques we have shared might help you to challenge and change unhelpful beliefs or behaviours that can create a set mind?

2. Are you a simplicity seeker? Can you ascertain why you are? What is taking up the space in your mental and emotional bandwidth? Could this be rebalanced?

3. Can you see in what ways you might unconsciously support unhelpful behaviours or beliefs? Do you use any kind of bias to confirm your ideas or beliefs? Or do you give yourself permission to act in certain ways through a seemingly, logical argument that is simply enabling an unhelpful behaviour?

4. Have you developed a system to be able to understand what your emotions are telling you? Can you be

comfortable when you experience uncomfortable emotions? Are you the problem-focused storyteller or the solution focused storyteller?

5. Do you use any of the 4 potentially unhelpful coping tools too much (denial, diversion, distraction, avoidance)? What could you do instead of over relying on these tools that would be beneficial both in the short and long the term?

6. How do you deal with guilt and fear? Would developing a new approach to managing guilt and fear assist in supporting your capacity to change? Do you have any specific fears that stop you from looking at yourself or taking accountability for your behaviour? Can you identify ways to manage them better if you do?

7. What emotional management do you use that works well? Can you see ways in which your emotions and how you handle them can prevent you from changing? What might help you and what might hinder you from using something like the pause, process and progress tool to manage your feelings? What are safe and helpful ways for you to feel and manage your emotions?

8. Are you an overthinker? What kinds of direction does your thinking take you in, positive, negative or fearful? Do you fill in the blanks with information that hasn't happened? Which tools and tactics could help you manage overthinking better?

9. Are there outcomes, things, roles or people that you can become unhealthily attached too? How could you ameliorate any negative impacts from this behaviour

9. Review of Insights into You

or what steps you can take to let things go more easily and compassionately?

10. What kind of thinker are you? Reflexive or reflective? How does your style of thinking affect your capacity for detachment? Or working with change? Or managing obstacles or block to change? Is this an area you could grow and improve in using some of the techniques discussed in both Book 1 and 2?

If you find these questions bring up difficult emotions, please pause and consider seeking support from a therapist or mental health professional.

Exercise: Memory Capture Revisited

Have there been any good moments today that you would like to capture and embed into your mind for use later when times might be tougher?

Take a pause to reflect now and make sure that you are starting to move into a space of experiencing rather than just having an experience. Or, familiarise yourself with this technique and use it at the next good moment.

Choose a moment from today, or recently, where you recall feeling good. Then answer the following:

1. What was happening at that moment?
2. Were you alone or were others there?
3. Which senses were activated (sight, smell, touch, taste, sound)?
4. What was the feeling in your body? Did it make you feel light, energized, relaxed, safe? Was this feeling all over or just in one place? Did you feel it in your heart or in your smile?
5. What did you contribute to making this moment occur? Or were you just a witness to it?

6. What thoughts did you have about yourself? I am being liked, recognized, heard, cared for, loved, etc.
7. What can you take from this memory to help you in tougher times?

Next Steps

If you have completed the work of Book 1, The Subtle Injury of Influence, and now the work of Book 2, I'm Getting There, your personal map of psychodiversity may be taking shape and expanding as you begin to fill in the details. You might now be more aware of the subtle influences that arise from experiences, relationships, and your social and cultural environment—and how these influences could impact your mental health and wellbeing.

Through the lens of self-compassion, you may have developed a deeper understanding that many of the things we do are entirely human and normal, but not always helpful. You may have started to identify what is working for you and what may be causing unnecessary stress or emotional harm.

You might also be recognising the value of having a supportive emotional coping strategy, one that serves both your short-term wellbeing and your long-term personal development. Along the way, you may have gained insights into how emotional responses, such as boredom, frustration, fear, or guilt, could become barriers to change. For example, boredom may disrupt the repetition required to help the brain form new habits. Impatience with slow progress, or fears of failure linked to self-worth, could discourage persistence. Guilt may reduce self-esteem and limit your capacity to take responsibility in a constructive way.

Over the course of the first two books, you've had the

opportunity to learn more about yourself. This ongoing exploration may be supporting the development of your own Adaptable Sustainable Psychology—a personalised framework that may help you respond to challenges in ways that minimise harm to others and protect your future self by reducing reliance on unhelpful or unsustainable coping strategies.

Part of building this framework includes managing your expectations and assumptions. Without reflection, these can lead us into patterns that feel overwhelming or counterproductive. In particular, the pursuit of perfection through constant self-development or the assumption that we must always be striving to become more can sometimes be as emotionally draining as not changing at all. This brings us to Book 3: Self-Improvement Burnout – When to start, when to stop.

Book 3 helps you locate that pivotal balance between pursuing growth and embracing the progress you've already made. It encourages you to sit with self-acceptance being ok to be you. Having introduced mindfulness in earlier chapters, this book explores the practice more deeply, including when mindfulness can be beneficial, and when it may not be the most appropriate strategy.

Using the self-awareness cultivated through Books 1 and 2, we explore how to sustain a sense of being "enough", of having done enough, and having enough to support your wellbeing. This core sense of self may become a reliable guide in determining when further change is required and when self-acceptance offers the more peaceful path forward.

In Book 3: Self-Improvement Burnout – When to start, when to Stop, we continue the journey of building your psychodiversity through the Adaptable Sustainable Psychology framework.

10. Alternative Self-Talk Tables

When you have spent so many years thinking badly about yourself or criticising yourself, it may be hard to think about how you might change this unhelpful self-talk. The following tables are designed as a quick guide to help you identify unhelpful thinking patterns that you may have developed and find and create new ways to think. The tables are here to support you in finding your own words and are not meant to be prescriptive or directive.

They may aid you in retraining your brain into more positive and supportive ways of thinking about yourself by reframing how you see things, how you talk to yourself, and how you talk about yourself to others. This could help you evolve a more secure foundation of higher self-worth, which may then aid you in seeing the times you need to be accountable, and the times others are negatively influencing you or even manipulating you and support yourself in changing and growing.

Remember that **perceptions power** our **emotions**. The way you perceive yourself can have a massive influence on how you feel, how you cope with life, and can even affect outcomes. The way you phrase things and set up a statement matters. For example, "I can't do it" means you can't do it. "I am going to give it a go and can cope no matter the outcome" might cost you more words, but it gives you encouragement, positivity, and uplifts you rather than putting you down. It can give you a soft place to land and try again if things don't work out, and may support your capacity to keep going.

Negative thinking, negative self-talk, or using negative language with both yourself and others in your everyday conversations could lead to:

- A lack of self-belief
- Low self-worth
- A loss of confidence
- Feeling anxious / guilty / fearful / depressed / sad / unhappy / dissatisfied
- Being unable to take chances and missing out on opportunities
- Loneliness or unhealthy relationships
- An increase of pressure on the self, which can lead to more mistakes
- Negative procrastination or impulsiveness

Maybe see if you've already experienced any of the items listed above. Or make a mental note of what could happen if you risk thinking negatively about yourself and being unkind or even cruel to yourself.

How to work with the alternative self-talk tables

The following tables have a soft reframe, advanced reframe, and self-coaching perspective. The words used might not be close to how you speak or exactly what you feel comfortable saying, but it may give you some ideas to play with.

A good way to use these tables is to notice when you feel

10. Alternative Self-Talk Tables

a strong, uncomfortable emotion and identify if it belongs to one of the following areas.

- Fear: What if – Comparison – Failure
- Guilt: Blame – I am responsible for everyone – I should
- Sadness: Hopelessness – Loneliness – Grief
- Powerlessness: Self-doubt – Why me? Why not me?
- Anger: Self-hatred – Not being heard/seen

Look through the tables below to see if any of the thoughts sound like you. When you find a thought that sounds like something you say to yourself or others, or resonates with the feeling you have, you can start by using the soft reframe, e.g. "I am learning to trust and back myself." If you're feeling comfortable, maybe use the advanced reframe and go from "I can't do it" straight to "I trust myself to have a go and cope no matter what."

The words used here are just a guide and might not be the same kinds of words or phrases you use. You are strongly encouraged to change the wording to something similar using your own style.

Look at the self-coaching column to maybe provide some extra support for yourself. Brain retraining can be slow, and it helps to be kind, supportive, and encouraging towards yourself to assist you as you remain on the path to change. Develop your own inner therapist or be your own best coach by actively giving yourself the help you need to go on. Maybe you take some time to work out what supportive and motivational approach could help you to continue to work on your thinking patterns until they evolve. Maybe seek some professional support with this process if that feels right for you. You may always have some negative thoughts or comments that come up in your mind, once they are programmed in they might not disappear sadly, but you can always meet them with compassion, care, and use a positive re-direct to move yourself into a line of thought that might help you, and cause you less harm.

You can use techniques from all the books in the Adaptable Sustainable Psychology collection to help you change your internal storytelling, such as the breath work, self-compassion, or mindfulness, to help you hear unhelpful thoughts. Use the affirmation training, the memory palace or the Emotional Freedom Technique to start training yourself into repeating the new thought patterns. Make it a daily practice. Ask friends and family to help redirect you if they hear you making negative statements. Trust that you are already in a process of changing and healing any unhelpful thinking, because you are, just by reading this book. Whenever you notice uncomfortable emotions or hear yourself making negative statements (either inside your head or to others) if you can, use the reframe straight away and adopt a self-coaching attitude that works for you. Rather than let the thought pass you by, change it on the spot or as soon as you can after you recognise it.

Maybe consider creating an attitude towards yourself that is based on compassion, kindness, and understanding, with the clarity that this negative self-talk is not kind to you and that you may have to keep working at changing or challenging this way of thinking or acting towards yourself.

1. FEAR: WHAT IF - COMPARISON - FAILURE

THOUGHT	SOFT REFRAME	ADVANCE REFRAME	SELF-COACHING
WHAT IF...	**WHAT IF...**	**WHAT IF...**	**WHAT IF...**
It has happened before. It happens to others. But this ... could happen. I'm too scared to ... because... What happens if... I will look stupid if I try. What will everyone else think? What if I don't make it?	I can learn to trust myself to cope with any outcome. I know where to find help if I need it. I can keep making choices. I can choose to back myself no matter what. I can choose to look after myself if I need to. Those who care about me will support me. I can support me too.	I know it could be tough, but I trust in my ability to find a way to cope no matter what. Thinking the worst will make me more scared and this is unhelpful. I can trust myself to make a clear, educated risk assessment using my knowledge and experience. I know there will be a way to get help if I need it. The people who matter the most will be kind. Those who are unkind are not my people anyway.	Fear is a healthy part of being human. It can keep us safe. But I know it can get out of control if it's not managed. We all have a fear response, and it takes mindful practice to settle it and become calmer. It's ok to have this feeling in this situation. Others who had my experiences would have it too. I can learn to support myself through this. It is normal to have doubts and fears, but I can choose to look after myself more kindly to help avoid becoming overwhelmed.

1. FEAR: WHAT IF - COMPARISON - FAILURE

THOUGHT	SOFT REFRAME	ADVANCE REFRAME	SELF-COACHING
COMPARISON	**COMPARISON**	**COMPARISON**	**COMPARISON**
Everyone else can. No one else makes mistakes. I don't look as good as that. I don't have that. I'm never going to be like them. I need to be/look like... Everyone is better than me.	I can learn to value my uniqueness. It is a fact that everyone at some point will make a mistake. Sometimes, it is a being human thing, not just a being me thing. I am willing to look at what I do have rather than what I don't. I am considering it is not helpful to think about myself like this. I could start to be more positive about being myself.	I can admire and like what others have and still be comfortable being me. It's ok to want things, but I can feel good about myself without them. I can own my mistakes because they teach me things. Everyone is learning all the time. I am glad to be me. I can grow and change, and I am grateful for what I have and who I am. It feels good to be me. I see what I have to offer and value this.	Others can make us feel that we are not good enough, so we buy their products and services. I can challenge this by being ok to be me. It is totally ok to want to improve things or change, but feeling good about myself must come from being content to be me without the extras. We are conditioned to think we need to be more; it will take time to learn to accept myself as I find that balance of growing versus accepting myself or my situation.

1. FEAR: WHAT IF - COMPARISON - FAILURE

THOUGHT	SOFT REFRAME	ADVANCE REFRAME	SELF-COACHING
FAILURE	**FAILURE**	**FAILURE**	**FAILURE**
I'll never succeed. I never get it right. I always screw up.	I can give it my best. I do many things well; I don't have to get it all right.	I am comfortable being me. A single outcome is not a complete representation of who I am.	Winning, losing, succeeding, and failing are about the ego needing an identity, not who I am as a whole person.
Typical me, failed again. I'm such a loser. No one likes a loser.	It's ok if it doesn't work out. I will find a way to cope.	I am more than ideas of success or failure. I can always learn more.	I have been told that being a winner or successful is the way to be liked or accepted. This is not an absolute truth.
I will lose respect if I fail. I succeed or I get laughed at.	I respect myself for taking a chance. I have good qualities; I don't have to be good at everything.	It doesn't have to be perfect or right. The fact I am having a go is enough for me. Everything shows you something. There is something good I can pull out of this, no matter the outcome.	This is old thinking that no longer serves me. I get why I do it because of the world I live in, but I need to update it.
I should have known...	I am learning to accept all of me. The attempt is as important as the outcome.	I trust myself to do my best and be kind to myself even if it doesn't work out.	It will take time to change these thoughts, but it is worth persisting.

2. Guilt: Blame - I Am Responsible For Everyone - I Should

THOUGHT	SOFT REFRAME	ADVANCE REFRAME	SELF-COACHING
BLAME	**BLAME**	**BLAME**	**BLAME**
I am always to blame. It's always my fault. It always happens to me. It's not my responsibility. I can't help it. Nothing ever goes my way.	Responsibility can be shared. Is there something useful I can learn here? I can keep making new choices. If I own it, I can grow from it. I believe I can make choices that will influence my life. I am willing to face my responsibilities with compassion for myself.	I need to step back and see what belongs to me, and what belongs to others. If I accept my part in this, I can change things. There are always positives and negatives. I get to choose which I focus more on. I am safe to take responsibility as I trust that I can cope with the outcome.	It may be uncomfortable taking responsibility, but when I do, I have more control to make better choices. Those who really care for me will respect my accountability and support me to change. Seeing things as nothing to do with me is unhelpful and limits my ability to improve my circumstances. It is hard to accept responsibility, but it is worth it.

2. Guilt: Blame - I Am Responsible For Everyone - I Should

THOUGHT	SOFT REFRAME	ADVANCE REFRAME	SELF-COACHING
I AM RESPONSIBLE FOR EVERYONE	I AM RESPONSIBLE FOR EVERYONE	I AM RESPONSIBLE FOR EVERYONE	I AM RESPONSIBLE FOR EVERYONE
I need to put everyone else first all the time.	I can find balance between what is mine and what is others.	I can be kind, compassionate, and understanding, but this doesn't mean people can take advantage of me because of their past or circumstances.	I know it can be easy for me to over give. My generous nature is a good part of who I am, but I must manage this to avoid burn out.
Others deserve more than me.	I can see myself as being equally important to others. There are times others come first, and there are times I come first.	I am responsible for my choices and actions. If others are not responsible for their choices and actions, this relationship is not sustainable.	If people abuse me, this says more about them than me. Abuse doesn't mean I deserve less. I cannot base my self-worth from cruel or violent acts.
Other people are more important than me.	Change is a process, something we all have a share in; everyone has a part to play.	I need to assess what the other person can do for themselves, what I can offer, what they can offer, and what we can achieve when we both self-manage and give equally.	When other people make me responsible for their lives or wellbeing, I need to question this. Is it my job or theirs?
I need to be the one to change.	I can work out when I need to step back and let others help themselves.		
It's up to me to do it for everyone else.			

2. Guilt: Blame - I Am Responsible For Everyone - I Should

THOUGHT	SOFT REFRAME	ADVANCE REFRAME	SELF-COACHING
I SHOULD	I SHOULD	I SHOULD	I SHOULD
I should do more. I should be better. I should know better. Everyone puts it on me. Everyone else is right; I am wrong. I am never right; other people know best.	I can work out when I need to do more and when I have done enough. I am allowed to share responsibility with others. My effort and openness to learn counts. I know myself best, and sometimes it's ok to reject other people's opinions. I am willing to learn to trust myself more.	There are always choices, and being able to work out when I can or need to do more, and when others can or need to more, is vital. We are all learning, we all make mistakes, I can take something good from this. The best relationships share care and accountability. These are worth finding. I can think about why people make negative comments. It might be more about their stuff than mine.	There is a balance between accepting that bad things happen and we can all do things that hurt others, and when others are unfairly blaming people for their own life history or situation. The quality I value in myself and others is being able to accept when things go wrong and working together to find a way forward. Sometimes we need to take a broader view of the situation. Looking at the past, at other people's behaviour, and the relative truths to work out what is going on and how we share accountability.

3. Sadness: Hopelessness - Loneliness - Grief

THOUGHT	SOFT REFRAME	ADVANCE REFRAME	SELF-COACHING
HOPELESSNESS	**HOPELESSNESS**	**HOPELESSNESS**	**HOPELESSNESS**
I can't change. Things will never change. Everything always goes well for other people. Good things never last. It's just one bad thing after another. My life is a sh*t show.	Neuroscience shows we can all change and the reality is life is always changing, even in small ways. I can choose to be a solution-focused storyteller. Other people make choices; I can too. Change is part of being human. Bad and good things pass, how I manage that is up to me. I'm choosing to focus on the good.	I believe I can influence my life, including how I see and cope with things. Change can be a choice, or it can be something that happens to us, and I can cope with either. The brain links one bad thing to another, but it does the same for good things too.	It's ok to say when things are hard, terrible, or painful. It's ok to know change can be slow and frustrating. But I can survive. I can cope. I can always choose what I focus most on. Sometimes the hardest thing I must do is find something to be grateful for, but huge efforts can give huge rewards.

3. Sadness: Hopelessness - Loneliness - Grief

THOUGHT	SOFT REFRAME	ADVANCE REFRAME	SELF-COACHING
LONELINESS	**LONELINESS**	**LONELINESS**	**LONELINESS**
I hate being by myself. All my relationships fail, so it must be my fault. I can't find anyone because I'm not good/pretty/rich/successful enough. People will judge me for being alone. Why would anyone want me? I don't like my own company, I can't stand being alone.	I am learning to enjoy my own company. Some relationships last longer than others, but I can learn from all of them. I am ok being me; someone else will be ok with me too. I am finding ways to be comfortable with myself. I am learning to trust in the qualities I have to offer others and to value myself.	If I cannot enjoy my own company, it might be hard for others too. I will learn to like my own presence. If thoughts come up that make me uncomfortable, I can change them. Rather than feel like a failure, I can learn from a relationship that did not work out and use that to help me make different choices in the future. By focusing on all my negatives, I reduce my confidence, making it harder to meet and connect with someone. I need to see the good too. I am able to learn how to appreciate, respect and even like who I am, when that happens I can enjoy being by myself and my own company.	What values do I want to share in a relationship with someone? If they only like me for my looks/money/job etc., then they are liking things that will change, not me as a whole person. Maybe that's not the type of person I want to be with. I am not helping myself when I hyper focus on the negatives. If I spend as much time and energy finding my positives, I will feel better and find it easier to meet someone who shares my values. Being ok to be alone and be happy in my own company is hard to achieve when others look so happy in love, but if I can find the joy in being with myself, I will benefit.

3. Sadness: Hopelessness - Loneliness - Grief

THOUGHT	SOFT REFRAME	ADVANCE REFRAME	SELF-COACHING
GRIEF	**GRIEF**	**GRIEF**	**GRIEF**
I will never meet anyone like that again. Who am I without…? I'll never love again. There is only one person/career/way of being I can't be me without…	It's ok to miss people; they are all unique. Each relationship/career offers an opportunity for discovery and growth. There is no limit on love and it's ok that it's different in different relationships. There are many sides to who I am. Different experiences let me learn more about myself.	Grief is an individual thing, and I can move through it at my pace. Learning to live again will help me heal. It is my choice if and when I open my heart again. But my joy in life does not have to be limited to one experience or one person. Loss hurts and grieving is a natural part of letting go. When we release something, we can make space for something new.	Moving through grief and loss is a tough process, and it's important to be gentle with what feels right for me in any given moment. Right now, I am not ready for something new, but things always change. I can be content as I am for now and open to that being different one day. Having an identity that relies on having one person, one job, or one situation will not allow me to explore more of who I am or who I could be.

4. Powerlessness: Self-Doubt - I Have No Choice - Why Me, Why Not Me

THOUGHT	SOFT REFRAME	ADVANCE REFRAME	SELF-COACHING
SELF-DOUBT	SELF-DOUBT	SELF-DOUBT	SELF-DOUBT
I can't trust myself. I can't make it. I'm not the type who succeeds. I'm useless. What would I know? I have no skills.	I am open to seeing that I can trust myself. I seem to have survived this far! I can feel successful simply from having a go. The outcome matters less. I am willing to recognise there are things I can do well. It's ok that I have my own unique set of skills, I don't need everyone else's skills.	By believing in myself, I give myself more confidence and a better chance to feel comfortable being me. I know if I keep putting myself down it is harming me. Being kinder to myself will help me on all levels. Comparing myself to others is unfair and unhelpful. I can choose to see my strengths.	There are lots of ways to feel bad about myself, and they can limit change, growth, and be discouraging. But I can choose how I speak to myself. I would never to talk to someone I care about so negatively. I am determined to learn to be kinder to myself. I will keep working on trusting myself, recognising that I always find a way to come through and have always had my own back.

4. Powerlessness: Self-Doubt - I Have No Choice - Why Me, Why Not Me

THOUGHT	SOFT REFRAME	ADVANCE REFRAME	SELF-COACHING
I HAVE NO CHOICE	**I HAVE NO CHOICE**	**I HAVE NO CHOICE**	**I HAVE NO CHOICE**
There is nothing I can do.	I can choose how I cope with this.	There is power and possibility when I choose to believe in myself.	The one thing I can always control is how I choose to see things and how I cope with life. If I am feeling things are impossible, I can find others who could help me see and feel differently.
It is what it is.	I can help myself, even if only in small ways.	I can change my feelings whenever I choose to see things differently and do things differently.	
Who am I to change anything?	It is possible for me to back myself up.	It is hard to accept something bad, but I get to choose how I cope. There are always ways to find help, even if it takes time or I have to keep looking for the right fit for me.	Sometimes our minds make us feel like there is no way out, no good thing out there or no good in ourselves. But this does not mean it is true. Our minds can get it wrong. Asking, is this an absolute or relative truth can help me.
Other people have the power, not me.	There are ways to creatively cope with difficult things.		
I'm stuck.	I am prepared to be committed to seeking solutions.	I can be patient and determined to wait for the moment where change can happen.	
There is no way out for me.			

4. Powerlessness: Self-Doubt - I Have No Choice - Why Me, Why Not Me

THOUGHT	SOFT REFRAME	ADVANCE REFRAME	SELF-COACHING
WHY ME? WHY NOT ME?	**WHY ME? WHY NOT ME?**	**WHY ME? WHY NOT ME?**	**WHY ME? WHY NOT ME?**
Everyone else always gets picked before me. I am never chosen/lucky. It always happens to me. I'm the one only this happens to. No one else has to suffer this. I don't get a choice. I have no value and nothing o value to offer.	I choose myself, and I choose to keep going. The effort means more than the result for me. There are things I succeed in. I can cope no matter what. Other people also have to deal with stuff. I am not alone in it. I can choose how I cope and how I let this affect me. I can see my own worth if I look past my self-doubt.	If I focus only on others seeing my potential, I can miss out on feeling good about what I can do and have done. Sometimes missing out can be a good thing, and it does not stop me from trying again. I can get more from the calm and easier moments if I work on being in them fully. Being present allows me to feel safer, clearer, and better able to make choices about what I focus on.	Being human and living in our pressured modern world can be very hard. It's understandable at times it can feel too much. But I can help myself at any time using what I know about me to improve things. How I see things has an impact on how I feel. If I am the victim, then I can't choose to change things. If I see the opportunity for growth, let go of self-doubt, and encourage myself kindly, I have a better chance to change. Not just my self-talk, but the environment around me too.

5. Powerlessness: Anger: Self-Hatred–Not Being Heard/Seen

THOUGHT	SOFT REFRAME	ADVANCE REFRAME	SELF-COACHING
SELF-HATRED	SELF-HATRED	SELF-HATRED	SELF-HATRED
I'm not good enough for… Why would anyone want me? I don't deserve… I'm ugly/stupid/useless. I can't stand myself. I'm not worth it.	I have more to offer than I appreciate. I am open to looking for my strengths. I can learn that I am as deserving as others. I am uniquely me and that's OK. I am willing to learn to like and value myself.	If I can see my own worth, then others can too. Everyone has good qualities and strengths. I need to put in the effort to see mine. Hating myself makes me feel awful and drives others away or allows them to use me. Allowing myself to like being me is a better choice. Being kind to myself is a good start to self-acceptance and knowing I don't have to be like everyone else.	It makes no sense to self-hate as I am always going to be me. I am always with me. I will find things to like about myself. The world sometimes makes us feel bad for being ourselves so they can make money or grab power. I choose to not allow this. It's ok to be different and have different qualities or strengths. Being chosen is not the only way to feel accepted or liked. I can feel accepted through respecting my individuality and being ok with it.

5. Powerlessness: Anger: Self-Hatred–Not Being Heard/Seen

THOUGHT	SOFT REFRAME	ADVANCE REFRAME	SELF-COACHING
NOT BEING HEARD/SEEN	**NOT BEING HEARD/SEEN**	**NOT BEING HEARD/SEEN**	**NOT BEING HEARD/SEEN**
No one ever gets me. Other people don't compliment my work/looks/efforts enough. The only way people notice me is when I am loud. No one values what I do. Why do others put me down?	I get myself, and that is enough. I can choose to feel good about myself regardless of other's feedback. I am committed to keep looking for people I can connect with. I value my efforts. Compliments from others are a bonus. Or I can ask for one if I need it. I can see when to back myself up and when I need help from others.	I choose to respect and value myself without always relying on input from others. If the people around me do not see my worth, then I may need to find new people. I can work out when feedback is valid or when the other person seeks to feel better by putting me down. Sometimes the comments may hold truth; sometimes it might be the other person's issue.	Relying on others to feel good about myself is unhelpful. When people feel bad, threatened, or stressed, they can take it out unfairly on others or use them to feel better about themselves. I need to work on valuing myself regardless of other people. I live in a world that uses fear and negativity to gain money and power. I can see through the agendas of others to know I am enough, I do enough, and have enough.

Acknowledgments - With Gratitude

I would like to respectfully acknowledge and thank all the individuals who have inspired, created, and contributed to our current body of psychological knowledge. This book draws on the brilliant work of many who have postulated theories, tested them, or created therapeutic techniques to help those in distress.

My deepest thanks go to every client I've had the privilege of working with. Each interaction has been a valuable learning experience, teaching me more about how humans are shaped by one another and the world around them.

I would like to thank my parents, who have provided a backdrop of consistent support. I am deeply fortunate and blessed to have been inspired by my mother's constant capacity for forgiveness and care, and by my father's determination to keep moving forward, no matter the obstacles.

I'm incredibly grateful to my dedicated, kind, hard-working, and funny partner, Andy. Knowing his love and support is there as a constant, and receiving his encouragement when things have been difficult, has made an enormous difference over the past few years.

To all my friends, thank you—particularly Talina, who has never doubted me and has been a steady stream of support, encouragement, and kindness. I'm also super grateful for my long-term school friends Kerry, Katie, and Laura, whose wisdom, humour, and compassion carry me through life's challenges. And to Jim, whose company has been one of the greatest blessings—offering nourishment, fun, learning, and the simple joy of sharing life.

I would like to express my gratitude and respect to my mentor and supervisor, Dr. Bruce Wilson, for his care and guidance over the years; to Helen and Alex for their generosity, intelligence, and skills in promoting this work; and to Kerry for her editing talents, positive support, and insightful guidance.

I'm extremely thankful to everyone at Author Services Australia who helped bring this book to life. Regardless of the outcome, I'm truly pleased with what we've created - thanks in large part to the brilliant, patient, and hard-working individuals who put up with my endless list of revisions.

My final acknowledgment goes to my first husband. While I lost you on the 12th day of the 12th month in 2012 – a day where so much of my world ended - I have from that awful moment been continually supported by the love we shared, the hope you gave me, and your constant belief in what I could achieve. I would not be who I am without you

www.ingramcontent.com/pod-product-compliance
Lightning Source LLC
Chambersburg PA
CBHW061727070526
44583CB00024B/3037